HowExpert

MW01132248

Color Blind 101

101 Tips and Stories to Understand, Embrace, and Live Your Best Life with Color Vision Deficiency

HowExpert with Kim Springer

Copyright HowExpert™
www.HowExpert.com

For more tips related to this topic, visit HowExpert.com/colorblind.

Recommended Resources

- HowExpert.com – Quick 'How To' Guides on All Topics by Everyday Experts.
- HowExpert.com/books – HowExpert Books
- HowExpert.com/products – HowExpert Products
- HowExpert.com/courses – HowExpert Courses
- HowExpert.com/clothing – HowExpert Clothing
- HowExpert.com/membership – Learn All Topics from A to Z by Real Experts.
- HowExpert.com/affiliates – HowExpert Affiliate Program
- HowExpert.com/jobs – HowExpert Jobs
- HowExpert.com/writers – Write About Your #1 Passion/Knowledge/Expertise.
- YouTube.com/HowExpert – Subscribe to HowExpert YouTube.
- Instagram.com/HowExpert – Follow HowExpert on Instagram.
- Facebook.com/HowExpert – Follow HowExpert on Facebook.

Table of Contents

Introduction:

Everyday decisions sometimes pose problems for me. Does this shirt match these shorts? Has the beef browned in the pan? Did that driver have his turn signal on?

Yes, I am color blind, but I rarely think about it. Consider it this way. I spend a lot of time listening to music and picking out the key signature, time signature, chord progression, and melody. I am always astounded when people can enjoy music but have no idea how to read it or replicate it on the piano or another instrument. I cannot imagine living that way, but most people without musical training do. That is how I am with color. I can appreciate it, but I will never, naturally, see it the way most people do. And, I am okay with that.

If that analogy does not jive with you, consider food. To some people, food is sustenance. We eat it to fuel, heal, and maintain. To others, food is an artform. Cheese comes is a gazillion varieties for a reason. Same with wine, pasta, and all other staples. Plus, the way vegetable are grown affects their flavor immensely. I can still remember the taste of my first fresh carrot unearthed from my own garden. It burst in my mouth like a sunrise; had no one told me it was a carrot, I may have guessed some savory dessert item. I imagine my color blindness is quite like store-bought carrots or living with only American cheese, but I am better off this way. It is what I know. I could not, however, live with limited food choices!

Most of you are probably reading this because you are color blind, so in this eBook, I will tailor my material to you. There is also helpful information and anecdotes for the relative of a color blind person or naturally curious. We are a mighty force, but sometimes we need help navigating the mundane decisions others take for granted. In this "how to," I will attempt to ease some of the tension you feel every day. I am hoping to inform, aid, and entertain you as we both celebrate and commiserate our color blindness.

As an American, my material will stem from my American and abroad experiences and will not comprehensibly cover color blindness in all countries. Several countries treat color blindness differently than America, but I will be using my "ethnocentric" knowledge to inform this eBook. I by no means intend to diminish another country, or even US state's, way of life, but respect all cultures. That being said, let's unite over our color blindness. Increasingly our world is open to those who deviate from the norm, so let us be a part of that powerful subculture!

Chapter 1: What Kind of Color Blind Are You?

Color Blindness from Behind These Blue Eyes

Do not be discouraged when strangers and acquaintances alike think they understand your color blindness because they read a posting online. Color blindness, while divided into a plethora of categories, varies from person to person. Even people diagnosed with the same condition will experience it differently. While we can find comfort in commonalities, it is important to approach each person as an individual, who sees their world from their eyes, not a textbook pair of eyeballs.

The color blind can also suffer from nearsightedness, farsightedness, sensitivity to light, glaucoma, and other eye conditions. In addition, we have other medical conditions, likes and dislikes, learning abilities and disabilities, and other factors that affect how we live with our condition. We need to be approached as individuals and not summed up by a medical diagnosis. Therefore, I will attempt to explain our conditions in generalized and personal terms below, drawing on what I have learned from behind these blue eyes.

Total Color Blindness: Seeing the World in Black and White

I have zero personal experience with total color blindness, but I have studied it mildly. I have upmost respect for anyone who lives with this condition. As a partial color blind sufferer, I could never completely understand your handicap or address its needs, but I will attempt to pay tribute to you by touching on your condition and hopefully providing some tricks, support, or other forms of help or reassurance.

Tip #1: People with total color blindness only see gradients of black and white.

Known as monochromacy, people with total color blindness see degrees of black, gray, and white. To remember this term, think of monochromatic photography, with its richness and beauty stemming from the simplicity of the array of black and white shading and contrast. Varieties of other colors appear in degrees of brightness. For instance, a neon yellow will appear brighter than a midnight blue. In order to communicate with others, the totally color blind often memorize items by their color. Sight, while limited, is still beautiful for the totally color blind.

Tip#2: The totally color blind can find a support group or system.

While a color blind support group would behoove any sufferer, the totally color blind need extra help and support with everyday and milestone decisions. Joining a group provides educational, emotional, and other methods of support. Just talking with others who suffer from this condition is beneficial. A quick Google search reveals several websites and support groups such as the Colour Blind Awareness group that provides links and articles as a launchpad for help. Remember, you do not have to go this alone!

Total color blindness is an extremely rare condition, but let us rally around those who live great lives with this handicap. While I do not think the totally color blind will get national airtime for a pride parade, I think general awareness and education can enhance their experience in our communities.

Partial Color Blindness: A Limited Rainbow

Like most of you, I was born with partial color blindness but did not know it until an older age. I think my life would have unfolded rather similarly had I not known about my handicap, but I am grateful for the gift of knowledge and the understanding it brought to those in my life. Let us take a look at how we can explain partial color blindness from a personal point of view so that an uninformed population can understand.

Tip#3: People with partial color blindness struggle to see certain colors.

Partial color blindness has several names and faces. This book will not address the technical names of each color blind condition or attempt to explain the inner functions (or lack thereof) of the eye and its cones and pathways. For more technical information, visit the American Academy of Ophthalmology (AAOP), the National Eye Institute (NEI), or another reputable medical source.

In layman's terms, the most common forms of color confusion are red/green and blue/purple. This means that varying shades of red and green and/or blue and purple are undetectable to the colorblind eye. For example, a panorama of autumn leaves appears in various hues of green, orange, red, and brown – or so I am told. While I experience the changing colors of leaves, I cannot see every hue. I can tell you precisely when the Red Maple will display its bright red leaves or the Sugar Maple will shed its yellow wonders due to years of observation, but I cannot see the shades leading up to their transformation and departure.

Tip#4: Use real-life examples to explain your color blind experience to others.

I use illustrations, such as the one above, to describe my color blindness because the technical terms lack the dimensions that personal depiction provides. It is the difference between a sphere and a circle. Medical terms elucidate on a two-dimensional level, whereas real-life examples are three dimensional. Try using your own stories to help your loved ones understand your experience.

Also, specific diagnosis holds very little relevance for me because I never completely mix up red, green, and brown or blue and purple. Maybe you experience this too. Instead, my eye does not pick up certain shades of green, especially in particular situations where lights may be low or the material of an item makes it hard to comprehend. A shirt in bright light may appear green to me, but in dim light it looks tan. Material matters too! I thought my velour bathroom towels were tan for years until my husband pointed out that they are a very light green. Taking the time to study the towel's color and compare it to other greens on different materials helped me comprehend the color beyond just trusting my husband's perfect color vision (he's 20/20 vision, too! Some guys have all the luck;).

Blue, in all its shades and splendor, is my favorite color, but sometimes I think purple is blue. The undertone of the shade of purple may influence my perception. For instance, some lavenders appear indisputably purple because of their pinkish undertone. Also, some shades of violet are obviously purple due to their underlying blue. I believe the pink undertone is often more deceptive to me, but there does not seem to be a cut-and-fast rule. Do you suffer from this too?

Some purples always masquerade as a true blue - like periwinkle, the most indecisive color on the wheel. While periwinkle falls under the color family of both blue and purple, often other people will agree that a certain hue of periwinkle looks primarily blue or purple. I, however, am left disagreeing with the majority and at a loss for matching it with other colors. Hence, fashion flub ups.

These real-life examples help to flesh out my personal color blindness to others; still, sometimes people need explanations in terms that apply to their own lives.

Tip#5: Use common color-disputed situations to relate to those without color blindness.

Perhaps you experience frustration explaining your color blindness label because your condition does not fit nicely in a category. Just remember that the majority of people have not experienced our condition and cannot relate to it by a medial explanation. Therefore, I usually explain it to the color-accurate friend or family member in a way they can understand.

Ask your inquisitor, "Have you ever argued with a spouse or friend over the color of black or navy blue pants?" It seems that the color-accurate world does not distinguish between these two colors consistently. This is completely hilarity to me because I distinguish these two colors invariably (or so I think). Depending on the light or material, everyday people think a midnight blue is a black or a black is a navy blue. Often, they ascertain the color by checking the label or holding it up against a true black garment. These are color tests that the color blind are familiar with and use on a daily basis, so try relating that scenario to a friend and see if they can translate it to your color blind condition. If the medical explanation, which contrasts our cones and pathways to that of the regular eye, only confuses the situation, comparing may benefit your relationship more than contrasting.

Undiagnosed Color Blindness: Defying the Odds

Some people live their entire childhood, or even life, not recognizing that he or she is color blind, and that is okay! It is easy not to diagnose the condition because most color blind people see color. I actually prefer the term color deficient for this reason; deficient implies that color is limited not missing. Perhaps this explains why color blindness may go undiagnosed.

Tip# 6: Most color blind people are partially impaired, not completely.

While statistics vary, an extremely liberal estimation presumes that partial color blindness tends to affect less than 15 percent of the population, meaning that certainly no more than 15 percent of the population suffers from this condition and probably less statistically. Additionally, it is widely recorded and accepted that color blindness is extremely rare for women, affecting 5 percent of the population in a liberal estimation. Further explanation on the gender inequality appears in subsequent chapters.

Tip#7: Color blind individuals may be closer than they appear.

I had never encountered another color blind female until I attended college and broadened my social circle. My Psych 101 college professor at the Pennsylvania State University asserted that 1 in 10,000 women are affected by color blindness. Next, he asked any color blind women to raise their hands or stand up. Astonishingly, three women in my Psych 101 class voluntarily affirmed their color blindness when he poled us. Our class size was large, but well-below 30,000 people; we defied the odds. Or did we?

Tip#8: Contemplate that you or a loved one has undiagnosed color blindness.

As word spread amongst friends and family that I was writing a "how to" book on color blindness, they began to share their personal struggles and curious questions about color blindness. Some individuals reacted with denial or anger about the condition. Several were truly compassionate, and others teased in kindness. A few commiserated by offering their personal stories. Unexpectedly, a couple people briefly questioned their own color vision.

One person offered a story that I continue to ruminate. This teacher shared that students had corrected certain color choices made on the job, namely referring to a purple pen as blue. Since this color confusion does not inhibit daily life, this teacher's fleeting suspicions warranted no further regard, but simply connected us for a moment in time.

Like my teacher friend and numerous others, slight color confusion may fly under the radar because it does not affect everyday life. In fact, these incidences may not qualify as color blindness. But perhaps they do? In such case, the number of "color blind" people may be much greater than the recorded number due to underdiagnoses.

Tip#9: Mild forms of color blindness may go undiagnosed.

Upon searching for online color wheel tests, I encountered a color blind blog featuring the Ishihara color test. This test will be discussed at length in a subsequent chapter, but for now understand that color-accurate people unanimously identify the same color-coded number in each pixelated circle test. The blogger enhanced the contrast between the dissimilar colors in the color wheel in order to enable the color blind eye to see the "hidden" number, or the number that only the color-accurate viewer can detect. The diagnosed color blind blogger was able to determine the number after the enhancement. However, I was not, proving that my color vision is more inhibited than hers. This experiment also led me to question how many people may have a milder, undiagnosed form of color blindness.

Tip# 10: Color blindness is mostly inherited.

If you have any color-seeing problems, inspect your family tree for a trace of color deficiency. Unless your color blindness is caused by trauma, severe mutation, or another under-researched explanation (such as diabetes or a medical condition that could affect sight), it should follow a predictable genetic pattern.

The X sex chromosome carries the gene mutation for color blindness. A male gets this mutation from his mother because she is either color blind herself or she is a carrier. A female must inherit the mutation on two XX sex chromosomes, and therefore, gets it from both father and mother. Let me tell you a little story to clarify.

At Christmas one year, a father gave his growing son a blue tie to match his blue belt and shoes. However, his mother, who was in charge of providing a blue shirt, gave him a purple dress shirt. Unfortunately, she thought it was blue and now his outfit did not match.

This silly story illustrates the genetic pattern of color blindness. In order for a male to be color blind, he only needs a mother to pass on the color blind gene, or purple shirt, on the X sex chromosome. Even though his father provides a perfect Y chromosome, or blue shirt, he cannot prevent his son from inheriting color blindness, or mismatching his outfit. In fact, the father's Y chromosome does not determine color blindness.

Tip#11: Women need two gene mutations to inherit color blindness.

In a sequel to the above story, a father bought his daughter a polka dot pink shirt and her mother provided a red stripped cardigan. Her heinous outfit even drew negative attention at the Valentine's Day Party. This is my story. With two X sex chromosomes, I needed to receive two color blind genes, hence the wild polka dot shirt and candy-canned cardigan. Females have less likelihood of receiving color blindness because they need the defect on both X genes.

Tip#12: Some color blindness is not inherited.

Complete color blindness, however, is inherited differently and affects men and women equally. Nonetheless, very few people have this condition, so it is comparable to a rare disease. Color blindness can also occur from trauma or other conditions, so this handicap should never be generalized but taken case-by-case. Can I get an amen from my color blind friends?

Chapter Review:

Your color blindness is unique to you. No matter what a doctor or friend has told you, you are the expert on your color blindness. Describe it to people in terms that feel accurate to you and that they will understand. Remember that people want to learn about your condition so that they can work well with you and reach common goals. You have something special to offer to your color-accurate friends, family, and coworkers and the beginning of that journey starts with your openness about your color blindness. In fact, some of your acquaintances may have a case of undiagnosed color blindness and could benefit from your insights. If your condition is received as a stigma, remember that you deserve better than that and react accordingly. I believe in you!

Chapter 2: Is Anyone I Know Color Blind?

The Color Blind Role Call

Primarily affecting males, but also surfacing in females, color blindness does discriminate. The gene mutation appears less frequently in females, along with anyone who is not non-Hispanic Caucasian. With only recent findings highlighting the ethnic probabilities in color blindness, our focus will remain color blind (pun intended) and without regard to ethnicity. With a broader focus, the ensuing chapters will highlight how males, females, and children manifest and live with color blindness, along with tips for each subgroup to thrive with their handicap.

Calling All Color Blind Men

Most people who are color blind are male. If you are reading this, you have probably been diagnosed either by a professional or a family member as color blind. Do not fret; men with color blindness live life quite the same as men without it. While your disability may interfere with a few job opportunities, primarily you'll have the same odds in this game of life as everyone else. With some humility, safety tips, and everyday solutions to everyday scenarios, you can find humor, strength, and peace with your limitations.

Tip#13: If your wife says you are color blind, she's probably right.

If your wife is anything like me, she thinks she is right about everything. It can be hard on a man to always be "wrong." Still, if your wife says you are color blind repeatedly, investigate it. Statistically, your wife's chances of being correct are at least double yours. Only with complete color blindness does your wife have the same chances of being affected as you. And that handicap is obvious. If your wife is bothered, but your color confusion does not affect anyone else (wink, wink), just take her advice the next time she wants to dress you (and then maybe she'll take yours for the undressing).

On a more serious note, if your color blindness affects other areas of your life, see your optometrist or primary care physician. If you are cleared of the accusation, you can go on your merry way. If you are color blind, you have the right to handle that information as seen fit. If you can perform well and safely at your job, you do not need to disclose your new information. However, if you encounter any unforeseen color challenges, you have a reason to pause before continuing said path. You never want to intentionally deceive your employer because your boss may have better insight than you. For more on careers, see the following chapter titled as such.

Tip#14: Undiagnosed color blindness may negatively affect yourself and others.

Like any illness or handicap, leaving it undiagnosed can cause unnecessary stress on a person and his friends, family, and co-workers. If you continually felt dizzy, you would visit a doctor. To not do so would put unnecessary stress on yourself that could lead to moodiness and/or serious diagnoses in the future. Thankfully, color blindness most likely won't progress, but knowing the beast you are dealing with will help you tame it quicker.

Color blindness borders danger when a job or task requires quick and accurate color discrepancy. My husband is an electrician who deals with dangerous situations daily. At hundreds of feet in the air, he cannot balk when determining a color. Worst yet, he cannot choose the wrong wire to snip when working on a "hot" or currently electrified item. It could cost him or his crew their lives. If he were color blind, he could make minor changes to ensure safe work practices. For instance, he could work exclusively on "cold" projects, find tricks to distinguish wire colors (they do not change often and usually have a pattern), and always practice peer checks which are standard for the business anyhow. Knowing about color deficiency would simply make a good electrician great by keeping him safe and working well for longer. Of course, the employer should be informed and have the final say on employment if danger is sensed.

Tip#15: A diagnosis may help your progeny.

On a less serious but more personal note, undiagnosed color blindness may affect how your progeny assess their color-seeing abilities. If a child knows that his father or mother is color blind, he or she is more likely to test his or her color-seeing capabilities. In a following chapter you will read about how challenging color blindness can be for a child. Maybe you experienced some challenges as a kid that would have made more sense had someone told you that you were color blind. No one likes to feel alone in their handicap, and if you are color blind, you bring a sense of relief to your color blind child. They may reject the whole idea for a long time, but deep down, they are happy to not be alone in their struggles. Plus, you can show them the ropes.

Color blindness affects men more than women and can cause serious work and relational problems if left undiagnosed. Visiting the doctor is the best way to assess your color capabilities, but even an online test would shed some light on your situation. If you are labeled color blind, it should not affect your current daily life. Any jobs that require complete color determination will test for accuracy, and a diagnosis will only confirm the truth. You have nothing to lose and everything to gain from humbly accepting that you may be color blind. Let us put the guesswork to rest. Who knows - maybe you are color accurate?!?

Calling All Color Blind Women

Welcome to the club! Ladies, we are a small, but mighty force. Although we have a defect on both of our X genes, we still look great in jeans! Most color blind women never meet another color blind woman in their lifetime. I sat in a psychology 101 class with 3 other color blind women, quite the anomaly, and never met them. Penn State University was too large to start small chat after class. Anyhow, you will probably never meet another color blind woman, and that is okay.

Tip#16: Your color-accurate friends are your secret weapon!

Ladies, your color-accurate friends are irreplaceable. Yes, most of the women you meet will not be color blind, but not all of the ladies will be friendly, either. So, if you find a friendly gal who understands your color limitations, stick with her. Let her guide you through your awkward puberty years, through your wedding day, and onto whatever your bright future holds. If you do not have a bestie to help you, stick with your mom or use your wits!

Tip#17: Professionals offer free services that can guide you through your female endeavors and milestones!

Women are expected to figure out their makeup, coordinate professional outfits, plan weddings, and accomplish a portfolio of unusual feats, especially for a color blind woman. These experiences can be simplified and even enjoyable if you use the help of free services. Sometimes you have to get crafty, but remember that professionals are getting paid to help people figure out their makeup and whatnot.

My wedding planning illustrates the use of several free, professional services. Since I was a teacher and had the entire summer off, I planned the majority of my wedding details within the two months preceding my August wedding.

First, I had to plan the flowers and cake well in advance. These items required plenty of color decisions. In fact, the only color I chose on my own was mermaid blue. Since I had a summer wedding, I could not just mix and match with brown (too fall feeling), and opted to visit the florist first. Now my favorite florist worked at the local grocery store and could not provide the consultation services I needed. However, a high-end flower shop offered its services for free. Upon entering the establishment, I planned on using their flowers for my wedding, so I felt zero guilt when I did not use them after discovering their outlandish prices.

The high-end shop helped me pick out a variety of roses in the yellow and peach family that complemented my mermaid swatch well. Always bring a swatch or picture of whatever item you are trying to match. With names like mermaid, establishments are not always sure of the exact color, and you cannot trust your eye (or you can, you confident mama).

Tip# 18: Tip generously or pay for high-end services when your budget allows.

Armed with the perfectly-colored bouquet options, I approached my affordable local florist, and she made my dream bouquets for less. Plus, she worked with the grocery's bakery to incorporate live flowers onto my dream cake. The cake's design I found online from a fancy bakery. My decisions factored in a tight budget, but if you have the money to spend, support your local high-end shops. Without couture shops, "free" and professional services would be limited. Still, either way, use free consultations for peace of mind on your big day.

With the cake and the flowers behind me, I focused on moi – the lady of honor. Typical wedding dress colors, such as white, ivory or champagne, mix well with all other colors. Plus, places like David's Bridal provide free consultations for shoes, tuxedos, and more. So, all I really had to think about was makeup. I visited the local Boscov's a week before the wedding. The nicest consultant scooped me up and made me look like the Queen of Sheba. Thrilled with her free services, I purchased the lipstick she had chosen and returned a week later for my wedding-day face. My makeup looked exquisite on my wedding day and at the expense of only a few beauty items and a tip. It does not even have to be your wedding day to make use of a makeup consultant. Be their dream customer and ask for help! Tip them generously or support them through major purchases. Do not go it alone, friend. Color blindness does not mean we do not love color. We do! We just need a little extra advice.

Women with color blindness need to lovingly accept help from friends, family, and professionals in order to accomplish their color-related milestones. While we may not like to ask for help around every corner, others are more willing to advise us than we think. While most things in life are not free, many built-in services will guide you with color decisions. The next time you face a color crisis, use your wit to accomplish your goals. You have got this!

Calling All Color Blind Children

This chapter will primarily address parents of colorblind children; however, an older and mature child may benefit from reading this chapter by his or herself. For more information that would directly benefit a teenage reader, please see other chapters of interest, such as "You Stellar Wardrobe."

Tip#19: Always believe your color blind child when he or she says something is the wrong color.

Color blind children face unique challenges. Observing my son growing up color blind has reignited some of my old emotions, namely frustration. If your color blind child says that a brown item looks red, believe him. Tell him that he sees it that way and that mommy or daddy sees it as brown. Help him to learn the correct color identification while validating him and warding off additional frustration. Compare it to the age-old childhood game of naming cloud shapes. Some people see dragons, others see ballerinas, and some see ships. There is not a wrong answer. But to a child with color blindness, telling them they are completely wrong about what color they see, seems like they lost the cloud game. There should not be any losers- just people with various perspectives. Children will eventually come around to accepting their handicap as they learn to navigate it, and it becomes less daunting.

Tip#20: Color blind kids should be encouraged to enjoy colors as best as they can!!!

At the top of his class in reading and math, my son, however, cannot identify every color. Nonetheless, he is obsessed with the rainbow. Perhaps seeing blue, indigo, and violet in succession gives him a good frame of reference and provides some order and peace to the world of color. I remember thinking the rainbow was a farce because three colors were practically indistinguishable. I had to take it on faith.

Still, color blind preschoolers and early elementary students love color-related games because they are so prevalent. Red light, green light can be enjoyed without seeing any colors, and it reinforces the concepts behind those colors, teaching basic symbolism. Color blind kids fit right in while playing eye spy since their classmates are also guessing the wrong items. Plus, eye spy can be modified to include items that start with certain letters or rhyme with other words. For instance, my family plays alphabet eye spy, saying, "I spy with my little eye something that starts with A."

Board games like Candy Land and Mastermind Jr. reinforce colors for color blind kids by giving them direct color comparisons. Sometimes a color blind person can pick out a color by comparing it to the exact color with which they mix it up. Compare it to how experts spot counterfeit money; they do a side-by-side comparison of the real and fake. Sometimes purple appears purple if I hold it up next to blue.

Some games that ostensibly do not revolve around color will still confuse the color blind child. My son and I both struggle with our version of Shoots and Ladders. The board alternates between different shades of green squares and makes it hard for us to distinguish which path to follow. Even my color-accurate kids sometimes get confused. I teach all of them, especially my color blind child, to follow other directives, like arrows and numbers on the board.

Tip #21: If your color blind kid gets emotional about his clothes, consider any color blind challenges he may be facing.

Fall shopping with my son caused a few meltdowns. Namely, he needed each outfit to include a matching superhero top and bottom. In addition to the cool factor, my son wanted all his outfits to match, hung up with their partner, and requiring no guesswork. Since he did not state his intentions explicitly, I did not pick up on his strategy until well after the fact. Had I not shared his handicap, I may have never recognized his purposes. Nonetheless, he persisted in exacting his will and way in a surreptitious manner. My little buddy is a budding con artist at age 6. I could not be prouder!

If your color blind child wants to streamline some everyday processes in life, like picking out clothes, cut him some slack. Help him organize ahead of time or simply buy everything so that it matches. Any time you can make life easier for your color blind child, opt to do it!

Color blind children just want to fit in. They will not embrace their uniqueness until they are older. Help your child make smooth transitions throughout his childhood by teaching him color differentiation in a manner that uplifts him. Always validate your child while helping him learn about his uniqueness. Find ways for him to feel proud of himself, color or noncolor related.

Tip#22: Tell authority figures about your child's handicap.

While I will discuss education and color blindness in another chapter, it is worth noting twice that communication with a child's teacher, coach, nanny, grandparent or any other authority figure in his or her life, is imperative. Color blind confusion could masquerade as misbehavior, and no child should be reprimanded for something that is out of his control.

For instance, a child who has reached a new level of autonomy may attempt to conquer a new challenge that involves distinguishing color. A child should not be reprimanded for choosing socks that do not match or picking an unripe tomato from the garden. Rather, the color blind child needs guidance. A nanny can safety pin matching socks together or a camp counselor can teach the child about ripeness of fruit by touch. Remember to inform authority figures in your child's life about his or her handicap so that your child can learn and receive grace when they make innocent mistakes.

Tip#23: Educate your significant other about your child's handicap.

Whether your color blind child lives with his or her biological parents or another parental figure, ascertain that his relationships run smoothly by educating your significant other. Parenting is tireless and sometimes color blind mistakes erupt into senseless debacles. To continue with the matching socks example above, a parent may not realize that a child did not do his laundry because it was too challenging with his color blind handicap. Instead of accusing the child of laziness or disciplining him with more laundry, teach him a new system for laundry. These sort of creative, loving solutions begin with an informed parent.

Disseminating this information is even more important in blended or multi-generational families. While biological parents often play a key role in the discovery of color blindness or perhaps suffer the same handicap, a step-parent or grandparent-in-law may lack the necessary knowledge for understanding their step-child or grandchild. Consider how these key players learn best to determine how to share this pertinent information with them.

If an adult learns best by doing, create an atmosphere where the adult and color blind child can interact with colors together. Perhaps a color blind child can complete a color by number while the step-parent watches. This will allow the step-parent to observe the child either choosing the wrong color or reading the crayon wrapping to determine color.

If the step-parent is skeptical, remove the crayon wrappings first so that the child cannot read the colors. Undoubtedly, the color-coded picture will not emerge unless the step-parent helps. Be mindful, however, that sensitive color blind children may experience a range of emotions, like embarrassment or frustration, if their picture does not turn out right. In a group setting, the child may look around at a roomful of red apple pictures, while theirs is just a hodgepodge of colors, and feel ashamed. Similarly, a critical authority figure must withhold criticism and offer help. Take emotions and personalities into consideration before engaging a color blind child and less-informed authority figure in a color-related activity.

If your significant other is a visual learner, consider creating a Power Point Presentation or finding an informative video. Perhaps graphs or a book will inform the visual learner best. Provide the visual learner with pictures or even analogies that stick with him or her long after the initial learning session.

Perhaps your significant other is a great listener – lucky you! Choose your words carefully and explain the handicap clearly. Your astute listener will pick up the information quickly through a conversation and maybe an easy quip like, "Take your time with color blind."

Remember that even adults need time to grasp unknown handicaps. Be open to answering lots of questions and presenting the information in a myriad of forms. Patience is key, too. If a significant other refuses to accommodate a child, remain loving and seek help. Perhaps the significant other does not need to assist the child in his or her handicap. Or maybe your significant other can bring the child to his or her doctor's appointment and witness the color blind test firsthand. Never give up!

Tip#24: Explain your child's handicap to his or her siblings.

Peers can be brutal, especially with siblings - where jealousy, competition, and other petty emotions thrive. My three children mimic my chickens in their pecking order. Instead of bleeding beaks and food guarding, my children tattle, tease, and torment. Any difference between the children that is not accounted for by age adds fuel to the fire. Of course, basic moral and character training through family, school, community, or religious activities teach children diversity, tolerance, and acceptance. To older and more mature siblings, explain your child's handicap.

My middle child is color blind and both his older brother and younger sister are mature enough to grasp the idea of his disability. They are quite young, ages ranging from 5 to 8. We had a sweet family moment at the pediatrician's office the day that my middle child was diagnosed. The five of us, the pediatrician, me, and my three children, huddled together on the patient's bench. With legs swinging, hair twirling, and noses running, we all took the Ishihara test. The comely, yet motherly doctor led us through a child's lesson of the color blind test. Each child lit up as he or she learned more about their vision and each other's abilities. Since that day of illumination, my children have been sensitive to their brother's needs, and the pecking order has stalled – unless food or television is involved.

Tip #25: Grow with your child and his or her handicap.

As a child matures and reaches adolescence, their color blind needs will change. Females may experience embarrassment with the increasing demands for color coordination, and males may begin to flounder in an area of study. Males may become self conscious with their clothing choices, and females may realize that certain careers pose unfair challenges. Encourage your teenager to take ownership of their handicap and find their own solutions. This process of trial and error will require a parent's oversight, so be available when things go awry. Gently redirect them or illuminate areas of struggle if they are in denial or resistance. With the help of a loving parent, a color blind teenager can learn to live independently with his or her handicap.

Chapter Review:

Men, women, and children struggle with color blindness, but at unequal rates. Each gender and age requires special efforts to thrive in daily life and areas of expertise or increasing responsibility.

Transitioning from a child with color blindness to an adult with the same deficiency requires effort on the part of the parents, friends, family, and individual. If we are to succeed in our endeavors, we need to accept help at all ages and acknowledge that our handicap will not biologically get better or worse, but our condition can improve with a good attitude, hard work, and education.

Chapter 3: How Can I Tell If I Am Truly Color Blind?

The Official and Unofficial Color Blind Tests

At the risk of sounding like a horrible comedian, there are some telltale signs that you are truly color blind. If you cheer for the wrong team or shout the wrong color, you may be color blind. If you serve raw food, you may be color blind. If you take forever getting dressed, you may be color blind. If you ask for lots of help while shopping, you may be color blind. If all of these and more are true, you truly are color blind.

The Unofficial Discovery

Before a medical diagnosis takes place, a color blind person typically experiences some sort of awakening to their condition. Whether a parent, teacher, friend, or the individual discovers the handicap, the person comes to terms with their limitations through a personal recognition and acceptance. While I cannot speak to everyone's experience, I will share my experience as a color blind person and a parent to a color blind child.

Tip#26: Often parents or teachers are among the first to suspect that a child has color blindness.

While some primary care doctors or ophthalmologists may screen for color blindness, this has not been the primary means of discovery in my experience. Both my son and I discovered our color blindness through everyday activities and the observation of caring individuals.

My kindergarten teacher alerted my mother to my condition, explaining that I read the color crayon wrappers before selecting which color to use. She suggested that my mother let the doctor evaluate my color vision.

Paying it forward, my mother discovered that my son was reading crayon colors and alerted me. After observing his coloring habits for a millisecond, I agreed with her diagnosis.

If a teacher, spouse, step-parent or other loving individual in your child's life suspects color blindness, say thank you and follow up with a doctor's visit. If your discovery stemmed from a faithful leader, it is time to say "thank you."

Tip#27: Awakening to one's handicap can be traumatizing.

For me, the teasing was relentless in Kindergarten. Classmates held crayon after crayon in the air, questioning me about their colors. Truthfully, I did not know. I stayed tight-lipped, not giving them the satisfaction of any answer.

As a kid, I did not want to stand out. Color blindness singled me out almost as soon as I entered a social learning setting. One of the first learning objectives is the identification of colors. I did much better at the application as I was a wiz at memorizing, but I could not tell blue from purple no matter how hard I tried. While the teacher understood and probably diffused the situation, I did not get it. How could I be adequate at every other task and yet have no ability to determine colors?

As disappointed and embarrassed as I was to find out I was color blind, it behooved me in the long run. Plus, I immediately knew that I was not just "stupid." I had a handicap. My son experiences the same feelings of inadequacy, but I am guiding him to slowly accept his handicap. With time and proper care, color blind people can overcome a rude awakening to their handicap.

The Official Discovery

While an unofficial discovery presents its own benefits, an official diagnosis validates the color blind person and opens up a world of information and support. Without an official diagnosis, the color blind person may wonder why he or she cannot perform certain functions or how to overcome their limitations. Official diagnoses also appear on doctor's charts and will help a child take ownership of their own medical needs as they mature.

Tip #28: The best way to tell if you are color blind is to visit your doctor.

The only foolproof way to officially diagnose color blindness is to take the Ishihara Colour Vision Test. This test consists of a series of dotted circles, each one containing a number or wiggly line. Either an online self-directed test or the doctor asks the patient to name the letter or trace a wiggly line, and a color-accurate person will be able to do that. However, the color blind may not be able to identify every letter and number. Which item he or she cannot identify will reveal his or her unique color blind diagnosis. While the online version is quick and convenient, a doctor can help provide guidance and instant feedback. If the online version revealed a color deficiency, I recommend visiting a doctor or optometrist to inquire about any lingering questions and to record your diagnosis in case of further investigation. Theories show that color blindness could be linked to other medical conditions.

Tip#29: Doctors may not offer the color blind test unless it is requested.

In continuation of my color blind story, my mother proceeded to take me to the doctor for a color vision test. The doctor initially refused to administer the test, stating that only boys were color blind. Always the trailblazer, mother insisted on the test.

The pediatrician held a circle test in front of my face and asked, "What number do you see?" Shyly, I replied, "A?" Clearly, I failed the test (or passed it, depending on how you look at it). He asked me to read other numbers and trace serpentine lines until he had verified what type of color blindness I had. Red/green and blue/purple, like my forefathers.

While coming to terms with my color blindness took a large step in maturity and did not happen overnight, the official diagnosis provided the springboard for such growth. Despite resistance and through the commitment of my teachers, mother, and myself, we were able to identify and treat this handicap in both myself and my son. Do not give up on getting the validation you or your child needs with their color blindness.

Spreading the Word

I am horrible at keeping secrets...especially ones that seem asinine. If the unraveling of the fib puts no one at risk, I might just slip. With serious secrets, however, I am a vault; I lived locked up about my color blindness for a long time.

Since I was diagnosed as a child and did not understand the shortcomings that surface in everyone's lives, I balked whenever my color blindness came into question. I see similar behavior in my son. As children, we both would rather ignore or deny the problem than receive negative attention. Ultimately, though, I learned to share my limitation, and obviously became comfortable enough to flesh it out in a book!

This chapter is experimental for me. I'll attempt to trace my "coming out" about color blindness while giving tips to help you do the same. Remember, everyone's journey is different, so sidestep any advice that does not speak to you.

Tip#30: It takes huge doses of emotional maturity to share your handicap.

While a parent or authority figure will oversee your color blind care during your childhood, around puberty or young adulthood, you are bound to encounter a situation where you must come clean about your color blindness. Remember, it is your decision to share or not to share. Friends and family members who surround you in daily life live with medical, emotional, and relational conditions and situations that they share with only selected, trusted people. If you are more comfortable circumventing the problem, do it. But if it cannot or should not be avoided, like in a job interview, learn how to open up in an emotionally safe way because you cannot control how others will react.

Tip#31: You do not owe it to anyone but yourself to explain your condition.

Admittedly, this statement is not entirely true. Some situations require disclosure of your condition for safety reasons. Also, your openness about color blindness may benefit loved ones, which I talk about throughout the book. Nonetheless, you do not have to share your condition with insensitive people. Sharing your condition should enhance your relationships and opportunities, not drive a wedge. Some reactions I have received when sharing my condition include:

1.) Oh, that is so weird. I had no idea that existed.

2.) You seemed normal to me. I would have had no idea.
3.) That must really suck. I feel bad for you.
4.) How do you do everyday things?
5.) How did you get this?

People fired out these callous exclamations and questions almost immediately upon learning about my condition. Can you imagine the lawsuits that would ensue if people reacted this way to individuals coming out about other things? Judge Judy would have fodder for a 24/7 show. Reread the list with another circumstance in mind, perhaps a missing limb or alternative lifestyle choice. Do these questions seem suitable?

Tip#32: You are an overcomer and can remain calm under fire

Before my fire runs too hot, I will back-pedal and explain why I am sharing these unsympathetic reactions. I have overcome each one, and you probably will or have already done the same! Since no one will thank you for remaining calm under fire, I am doing it today. Thank you for overlooking people's ignorance. Thank you for not explaining your condition to people who will never really listen and always think you cannot see color. Thank you for doing everyday things even though others react like you have a foreign, terminal illness. Your gift is emotional intelligence and you can unwrap it in any situation to release peace and production. You have overcome the inquisition!

Tip#33: Find a color blind "community."

While spreading the word with color-accurate friends and family acts as a milestone for emotional maturity and security in your relationships, color blind friends offer support that others cannot. If you find yourself struggling with everyday challenges, ownership of your handicap, or lack of support from your cohorts, search for a color blind community near or far.

Tip#34: Consider in-person and online support groups.

The easiest way to join a casual color blind support group is online. A simple Google search will reveal online color blind groups in which you can share your condition with other color blind folks. Beware to follow basic online safety rules, especially if you are still a minor. If you feel vulnerable at any point in time, find a live support group or close friend to confide in. Online support groups are for occasional and lightweight assistance. Handle any substantial needs with a professional or trusted ally.

Live support groups exist, but you have to be willing to search for them. Local support groups for color blindness are far and few in-between, but it is worth a shot if you like in-person interaction. Your local library, optometrist, or even vision rehabilitation group could point you in the right direction. Ascertain the group feels safe, meets your needs, and works into your schedule if you intend to attend regularly.

Tip#35: Start your own color blind support group.

If you cannot find a local color blind support group, start your own. With a few friends, central location, and basic discussion topics, your group can thrive with relatively little effort. Advertise at a local market, church, or school or choose to market online through a Facebook page. Be careful to market only to your community and never meet an unknown online friend alone or in a private setting. For the student, advertise at school, and for the elderly, advertise at the senior center. It may take a little more effort, but creating your own color blind support group may provide the encouragement you and others need.

Chapter Review:

While color blindness affects our sight, we cannot see it. This parody presents confusion for the child, or even some adults, when they discover that they struggle with color differentiation. After the unofficial recognition of the handicap, a doctor's official diagnosis can allay fear, frustration, embarrassment, and a wide array of negative feelings a newly informed color blind person may experience. Brazen individuals may rise about their color blind challenges without heavy assistance, while the more sensitive or those with severe color blind handicaps will benefit from a support group. Regardless of how arduous the journey may be, we will all prevail and learn to thrive with our color blindness, hopefully laughing along the way!

Chapter 4: Will Color Blindness Affect My Everyday Life?

Shopping with Color Blindness

I love to shop. Call it retail therapy if you like, but even my Goodwill purchases give me a euphoric high. Maybe you share this enjoyment, or perhaps shopping is a routine deal or a necessary evil. Either way, it poses unique dilemmas for us, the color blind. Drawing on about 20 years of shopping, I will share the tricks of the trade for the color blind. I hope the following witticisms and instructions infuse your shopping with joy and ease!

Food Shopping

We spend a large percentage of our life shopping, especially for food. With a wide array of healthy canned, frozen, boxed, and bottled foods, most food shopping items do not present a predicament for the color blind. Nonetheless, fresh foods often keep me scratching my head or asking for help. While sell-buy and expiration dates provide guidelines on meats, cheeses, and other dairies, fresh produce lacks such indicators and requires extra attention. Let the following tips and stories serve as a guide.

Tip #36: When life gives you lemons, make sure they are yellow.

Picking out produce poses challenges for the color-accurate and color-blind alike. However, fruits and vegetables do not come with color labels. So, unless you are shopping with a friend, you need some extra strategies for selecting fresh, ripe produce.

Tip#37: Wake up and smell the fruit!

Yes. Be that person! The person who looks like he is conducting a science experiment in the produce aisle. Do not just smell the fruit; knock on it, squeeze it, and anything short of tasting it – that would cross a line.

Do your research for each type of fruit, so you know what you are looking for. Melons need to smell sweet. Many of them are not going to ripen off the vine. Watermelon should sound hollow. Avocado and peaches should feel tender to the touch. Also, many fruits and vegetables are quite forgiving, so remember that bananas, tomatoes, and other staples will ripen over time and with each other. Be careful at home to store these fruits properly, as bananas and peaches may overripen without your noticing and that is the last thing you'll want to smell or taste!

Tip #38: Be berry careful.

Berry picking is a wholesome, healthy, and relaxing activity for the entire family, unless someone is color blind. Then extra precautions are needed. For instance, on my honeymoon, my husband and I dedicated an afternoon to blueberry picking. Equipped with crates upon crates, we sauntered down row upon row of beautiful berry bushes. Our wedding worries melting away in the hot August sun, we whispered sweet nothings through the branches and dreamed of blueberry pies, cobbler, pancakes...

After an hour or so of picking berries, we weighed the collection and paid the owner. Delighted we stowed away our berries in the freezer and later transferred them to our home's freezer to use for a pop of summer when the weather began to fade. Only we couldn't wait. Like Goldilocks, we sneaked a taste here and there, and found some were too sour, too small, and too purple!!! I had picked almost exclusively purple blueberries that would never ever ripen. Our freezer contained pounds of purpleberries. After a hearty laugh, we decided to mix them into the blueberries when we baked, with lots and lots of sugar and lemon extract. Next time, I will wear a blueberry-colored shirt as a guide for berry picking!

While fresh produce presents the most challenges to the color blind shopper, other food items wage war in the kitchen. We will look at the challenges of everyday cooking later in this chapter. For now, let us move on to another aspect of shopping – clothes!

Your Stellar Wardrobe

First and lasting impression often rely on a well-groomed appearance crowned by dapper outfits and accessories. Unless someone else does your shopping, you must find ways around your color blind deficiency in order to select and maintain presentable attire. I am here to tell you that this is not out of our reach or realm.

Even without concerted effort, we can implement a few routines and rules that allow for shopping and laundering freedom and fun.

Tip#39: Release any hard feelings towards those who previously ridiculed your outfits.

Choosing your wardrobe may seem daunting, especially if someone has pointed out your mismatched colors before, but being color blind and fashionable can go hand-in-hand. First off, let go of any hard feelings you have toward someone who made fun of your color choices involving clothing. Whether they meant to hurt your feelings or not, they are not worth your time and energy now. You have a great wardrobe to acquire and maintain!

If the mockers are still involved in your life, turn a deaf ear to their opinions. After you follow these shopping tips for the color blind, you can parade your stellar wardrobe down their catwalk or chose to take a higher road. Dressing for success will not only silence your critics, it will bump you to the next level of confidence at work, home, and around town!

Tip#40: Know what clothing *you* like and be confident!

Shopping as a color blind person starts by following your natural, wonderful instincts. Color blindness does not exclude your from have opinions as far as fashion is concerned. If you have never considered your style type, taking a short online quiz could reveal some telling results. Easier yet, walk through the mall with an open mind and enter the first store that speaks to you. Bypass any internal struggles by pretending you are on "What Not to Wear." Acting like this is someone else's narrative will melt away your insecurities. Have fun and pretend you are ten times more confident than your usual self.

If you already have an established style, contemplate two things: 1.) Does this style work for me and my color blindness? 2.) Have I been limiting myself due to my color blindness? If the answers expose a need for revamping, reread the previous paragraph. If you are already styling, start by selecting stores, catalogs, or websites that display the sort of clothes you love and need. Whether you are starting all over or picking up from where you left off, remember to be a confident shopper.

Tip#41: Let the experts do the hard work.

Taking tips from the experts is not a sign of weakness; it is a sign of wisdom. Regardless of where you are shopping, color-accurate people have already done the hard work of sorting, matching, and designing outfits. Make use of their services and save yourself time and energy. This is especially important if you have a specific objective. For instance, if you are in a hurry to select appropriate work attire, leave most of the work up to the experts.

Tip#42: Brick and mortar stores provide real-time interaction for quick results.

In brick and mortar stores, scan mannequins for looks that you like or see how the store has naturally paired items. Staying within the same brand for tops, bottoms, shoes, and other accessories will give you a seamless look that is more likely to blend not just based on color, but also on style. And do not be afraid to ask questions. Yes, you will get skeptics. I know I have! Since my color deficiency is a blue/purple confusion, less people are aware of my condition. After checking the sales tag for the clothing's' color, sometimes I am still unsure of the shade. I have asked fellow shoppers if certain shades of purple work together. Usually they look baffled initially. I have even had suspicious co-shoppers look around as if searching for a set crew for "Candid Camera." More typically, however, you'll notice the helpfulness of strangers. And if you are gregarious like me, it gives you a chance to spark up a new conversation. Bottom line, you should get a clear answer and/or a good story to share at your next party.

Tip#43: Catalogs and online shopping offer low-stress circumstances.

Catalog or online shopping is ideal for matching sundry outfits in a hurry. I used to be obsessed with the dELiA*s catalog as a teenager. My friends teased me about my monthly mad dashes to the mailbox. For a color blind teen with a lot of flare and interest in fashion, dELiA*s took the guesswork out of looking unmistakable me. Each page popped with clothing, shoe, and accessory matchups, along with references to other pages where the coveted items appeared in a different look. Today, online shopping can provide the same comfort and ease to color blind shoppers. With Pinterest, Instagram, Facebook, and more, you can find ways to expand your wardrobe without risking a major fashion flaw, and all from the comfort of your couch.

Tip#44: For a unique look, consider fashion choices that aren't based on color.

If you desire to be original in your outfit choices, try focusing on patterns, texture, jewelry, cuts, and shoes. So much of fashion has nothing to do with color, and you probably see the possibilities better than your color-accurate friends! Often, I will select a themed outfit, such as nautical, preppy, or classy, and complement it with my distinctive take on accessories. I still recall a leather Roxy watch that encircled my wrist throughout high school because I insisted on a road trip to acquire the timepiece. As trivial as it may seem, that lone accessory enhanced every look and decreased the guesswork in my daily routine. For men, consider selecting ties, shoes, cuff links, and more that distinguish you from others. A singular versatile item can inspire a plethora of outfits and streamline your accessorizing routine.

Tip# 45: Make it pop!

If you want a no-fuss rule of thumb: check this out. Center your wardrobe around black, white and gray – colors you cannot confuse. Then add one pop of color, like a stripped red tie, royal blue belt, or a pink dress shirt if you are feeling bold. People will comment on how they love the *colors* in your outfits, but really they are just noticing it because you have made it "pop." This is how a color blind person sheds their misnomer.

Tip#46: Do not be discouraged if you do not always match; people love you, for you!

Additionally, remember that a flub-up is not the end of the world. In fact, if you have kind, loving, accepting people surrounding you, they will most likely not mention a small fashion faux pas.

My husband is this way. Yes, I know, lucky me! But at first, I was furious with his indiscretion. Years after my bridal shower, my husband and I were reminiscing over photos from the event. Somehow it surfaced that my skirt and shirt did not match. I was appalled! Not only was this event a milestone in my life, I had worn that same outfit, one of my favorites, to a myriad of events during that stage of life.

After getting an earful, my husband assured me that I looked great in the outfit, and no one cared that it did not match. The truth is, he was right. I needed to recognize that my handicap gave others and myself a chance to extend grace, even on a topic as inconsequential as fashion. Trying not to be oversensitive about your color blind embarrassments will enhance the quality of your relationships.

Tip#47: Organizing your closet and dresser will pay off dividends.

Whether you are sorting well-loved clothing or new purchases, resist the temptation to mix them all up quickly in your closet or dresser. A little organization will go a long way.

Use a Sharpie to write the color from the sales tag onto the washing instruction tag. Now you have a permanent reference that won't wash off or harm other clothing. Next, hang clothing as outfits to ensure you pull off the look you wanted. Tired of the same old look? Using your tags, organize clothing by color. Now you can use your knowledge to create new outfits.

Tip#48: Have an efficient laundry sorting system.

To avoid a Paddington Bear mistake (he turns his inmate's uniforms pink), separate lights and darks ahead of time. If you have the space, designate a laundry hamper for white clothing only. For severe color limitations, preventing color bleeds in the washer is your number one priority. For more milder conditions, like mine, sort your laundry as needed – mine is sorted heavy, medium, handwash – but leave enough time to attend to your laundry. Although my colors are not previously sorted, I always group colors carefully when starting a load.

Setting aside previous fashion mistakes, enter your shopping experience with confidence. Once you have established your style and objective, do not be afraid to ask for help. Use mannequins and other visual aides to help guide your outfit choices. Reading clothing labels for color will assist you as well. If you cannot see it, you can still read it! For a one-of-a-kind look, uncover fashion choices that aren't based on color. With new or old clothes, organizing your closet and dresser will streamline your morning routine and increase your chances of looking put together. Additionally, sorting your laundry will prevent color bleeds. When all is said and done, however, remember to extend grace to yourself when an outfit or load of wash goes awry.

Transportation for the Color Blind

Staying Safe While Driving

Unless you are sporting a color blind bumper sticker, recognize that other drivers are completely unaware of your handicap. While you accidentally run a yellow light, tailgate another driver, or misread a road sign due to your color blindness, remember that other drivers might become angry.

Tip#49: Stay calm and drive on! *Or get help if dangerous mistakes are commonplace.

Whether another driver is angry, or you are frustrated with an unsafe situation your color blindness informed, staying calm is the safest option for in-the-moment mistakes. Unless you were in an accident or the police are involved, do not pull over for an enraged driver. Road rage is a serious issue, and explaining your condition will not help. Instead, read on for tips, and seek medical or driving assistance if unsafe mistakes are commonplace.

Tip#50: Memorize the traffic light pattern and other driving directives.

Orange, yellow, green: the colors of a traffic light for some color blind people. I first noticed this discrepancy well before I was of driving age. Elementary schools often use this "easy" traffic light system as a behavioral self-control tool. Most children adapt quite readily, considering the popular game "red light, green light," and the relative ease of identifying colors. Nonetheless, the color blind kids are left to their ingenious ways to quickly recognize sequencing and memorize nonsense (orange= red, white=green).

But on the road, the stakes are a bit higher. Thankfully, this typically is a minor problem; however, on a tired day or for the severely color blind, it poses a major risk. Having recognized this hazard, pigment has been added to enhance the colors for us. If you think your color blindness has improved, it may be that the world is finally seeing things our way!

Some countries and states have ditched the vertical traffic light setup and use horizontal lights or even shapes to organize their stop, slow, and go sequencing. Fortunately, this nonconventional setup confuses not only the color blind but also tourists, so you will not be alone. Go ahead and ask for help. And if the vertical pattern throws you for a loop, be sure to check with the locals as well.

Tip#51: Employ defensive driving.

While every driver should employ defensive driving, such as looking for reckless drivers, color blind drivers need an extra layer of awareness. Especially, we need to observe any physical damage to cars or roadway equipment because it can impair our ability to see color. For instance, I almost rear-ended a sedan whose brake lights and turn signals were encased by foggy orange plastic. As the sedan barely slowed to execute a right-hand turn from a highway into a convenience store parking lot, I slammed on my brakes, missing it by inches. Upon quick inspection, I noted that hazy encasements hid her brake lights and turn signal. Our best defense against improperly maintained cars is to avoid them. If I had been more observant, I would have switched lanes prior to the near accident.

Tip#52: Do not sweat the driver's test.

While rules and regulations on color blind drivers may have changed in the past 20 years, I do not recall any mentioning of my handicap at my driver's test. For me, the hardest part of driving remains parallel parking. If you can perform the necessary skills to pass the driving portion of your test, color blindness will simply affect a few color questions on the written portion. This information can easily be memorized, and I do not remember any difficulties. If you prefer further assistance or updated information, ask the DMV for more information regarding color blindness and driving. Do not hide your handicap if it puts you or others in peril. Otherwise, enjoy the open road!

Oh, The Places You'll Go, Public Transportation Abroad

Navigating a new roadway or metro system is difficult for everyone, but especially the color blind. We need user-friendly maps that are not always readily available. I have run late for job interviews, college courses, and other important engagements due to non-color blind friendly transportation systems. While your hometown, whether you are settled there or brand-spanking new, will become familiar to you over time, traveling abroad poses some serious safety concerns and transportation challenges for the color blind.

Tip#53: Never travel alone, abroad.

While this is a helpful tip to anyone who plans to travel abroad, unknown territory is especially tricky for color blind travelers to navigate. If you are on a work trip, stick with the group or ask for an assistant to accompany you. If you are a tourist, consider traveling with a group or partner. Perhaps you are a study abroad student; stay with your host family. Once you have the method of transportation and lay of the land figured out, then consider traveling alone if necessary.

Tip#54: Learn the transportation system immediately.

Whether you are visiting a city in your country or abroad, familiarize yourself with the primary public transportation method. Even if you have managed to travel with a friend, coworker, or family, still manage to carry maps and navigate well. When traveling in France, my friend and I inadvertently got separated from our tourist group. We ended up map-less in Notre Dame, quite literally praying for a miracle. Due to our ill preparation, we were at a complete loss. Thankfully, our tourist bus zoomed by and we were able to catch up with the group, but only after what felt like hours of panic. Color blind or not, learn the transportation system upon arrival. If the colors confuse you, circle the routes that lead back to your hotel or another safe location, like the police.

Tip#55: Opt for a cab, taxi, Uber, or other private transportation option.

When the metro or subway is too color complicated, chose another method of travel. For example, I traveled with a college group to Europe in the summer of 2006. When in Rome, we did as Romans did. We used a frenetic cab driver. Seriously, the roadways in the suburbs and downtown Rome are massively entangled and non-systematic. Plus, the drivers rarely use turn signs but rather hand gestures both appropriate and vulgar. Although not perfect, using private transportation erases the need to master color-coded maps and roadways and increases the enjoyability of your trip!

Tip#56: Study the metro system before using it.

France, England, and other European cities travel by color-complicated metro systems. Subways involved crisscrossing green and orange pathways, often indistinguishable to the color blind eye. Nonetheless, most rails had a number, direction (north/south or east/west), or detailed outline of cities at which to stop. Studying the map ahead of time allowed for ease of travel. Just remember to "mind the gap" when riding the tube! It is color neutral.

Tip#57: Use GPS.

While a traveling buddy is optimal, sometimes technology sticks closer than your buds. As long as there is a signal and you are not traveling a remote, uncharted location, GPS should get you where you are going (and with a proper accent). I have never used GPS abroad, but often it leads me down winding backroads in my country without fail.

Tip#58: Change your phone's color filter.

To get optimal performance out of your GPS or digital map, alter your phone's color settings to your preference. iPhone and Android now offer color blind users color palettes based on their deficiencies. In your settings, select the color blind option that fits you, along with the brightness or hue you prefer, and voila – your phone reflects the world as you see it!

Whether you are mastering your hometown roadways or complicated transportation systems abroad, traveling safely is not beyond the scope of the color blind. We pass our driver's tests, drive defensively, and navigate public transportation every day despite our handicap. Employing the help of others and technology enhances our opportunities to travel confidently and safely. Oh, the places we'll go!

Benefits and Hurdles with Learning

Knowledge is the building block of life. From the day we are born, we engage our senses in a lifetime pursuit called learning. At home, in school, and on the street, we observe the world and people around us, drawing conclusions and categorizing information. Everyone learns and categorizes differently, but we, the color blind, face unique benefits and hurdles due to our limitations. Let us explore our extraordinary learning process below!

Color Blindness and Learning on the Go

Color blind children and adults will employ their smarts in everyday situations to overcome their limitations. We can learn to accomplish almost any task with a little ingenuity and determination. Sometimes our weakness may prove to be a strength when our refreshing point-of-view breathes new life and perspective into a challenging situation.

Tip#59: Find alternative ways to approach color-related problems.

While many pastimes, assessments, and other activities summon our color-distinguishing abilities, we can beckon alternative approaches in order to engage effectively. For instance, puzzle-making is a classic, wholesome pastime - and a pain in the neck for color blind people. While most children and adults match up colors to connect puzzle pieces, the color blind person looks at the pieces' shapes, patterns, and placement within the puzzle at large.

Recently, my family set out a puzzle for a long winters' day. My husband and two color-accurate children selected puzzle pieces based on their matching colors. Recognizing the overwhelming brown and green color scheme, my color blind child and I implemented a different approach; we started by looking for straight edges and making the frame. Then we looked for patterns to connect and shapes that had complementary fittings.

My oldest and most competitive son chided, "Mom, those are different shades of green." Exasperated, he banned me from certain sections of the puzzle. Nonetheless, the only missing pieces – the nose of the cheetah, the tip of the toucan's beak, the lost blade of grass – emerged in my hands. I believe I could see the pattern through the colors. My family glanced at me inquisitively. How did the color blind lady find the missing piece?

Color Blindness and Learning at School

Color blindness will affect the formal education process and could lead to unfair scoring and profiling if accommodations are not set in place. We must inform the educators of our handicaps before they can inform us.

Tip#60: Consider a 504 for your color blind student.

Please parents, tell your child's teacher about his or her handicap. You have no idea how much grief this will save both of them, especially if your child is shy like I was. While I did not have a 504 or any form of specialized education plan, my informed teachers were able to make accommodations and the uninformed were not. A 504 will follow your child throughout his educational career and prevent their handicap from falling through the cracks.

Tip#61: Be your child's advocate if a dubious situation arises.

Respectfully engage with authority when a dubious situation arises. While most educators want to rally for your child, some teachers will dole out unfair treatment without considering individual conditions. For instance, my brother's elementary school teacher accused him of not correcting his writing mistakes. She directed the class to correct all mistakes marked in red ink. My brother only saw black ink and assumed he was in the clear! With my mother's intervention, the problems was cleared up.

Similarly, I attempted to cheat on a fifth-grade map test. With all the explorers' paths marked in blue or purple, I could not determine where they had traveled. Unfortunately, my scribbled answers dripped down my sweaty arm where they had been meticulously placed, and I received a lower score that day. Being penalized for something out of my control was not okay, but my diffident behavior left the injustice unrectified.

Tip#62: Commodify your color blindness.

You have suffered enough injustices at the hand of color blindness, so when an opportunity to exploit your handicap arises, take it. Color blindness is a misunderstood anomaly and researchers need participants. In college, my color blindness paid off, literally. In a college experiment, researchers sought out color blind students, especially females, to comment on new topographical maps for the color blind. I made some much needed cash and helped improve map reading for color blind people everywhere!

In school and on-the-go, color blind folks learn in well-known and yet-discovered ways. We employ resourcefulness when our color blindness inhibits us and commodification for our benefit. Remaining honest about your or your child's color blindness will only enhance the learning experience.

Chapter Review:

Color blindness reaches its insidious influence into all aspects of everyday life. While its limitations are limited, simple tricks of the trade help ease shopping, traveling, and learning. With concerted effort to label, prepare, and ask for help, the color blind person will thrive in everyday situations. And while sometimes our handicap may seem unfair, do not forget to enjoy the everyday blessings – like stopping to smell the roses, to hear the birds singing, and to embrace a loved one.

Chapter 5: Does Color Blindness Affect My Career Choices?

Yes. Unfortunately, color blindness is a handicap and must be taken into consideration when deciding on a career. I, intuitively, chose a career that did not involve color differentiation and would imagine that most color blind people would not want to put themselves or others in a compromising situation by choosing a career for which they were not fit. That being said, color blind people thrive in almost every line of work, especially when adaptive equipment is used properly. Let us take a closer look at the career outlook and adaptations for us, the color blind.

Most Common Careers

Tip#63: Color blind workers thrive in environments that do not rely on color differentiation, especially when safety or health is involved.

Some top-notch jobs for the color blind include civil engineer, teacher, lawyer, nutritionist, and many more. These jobs rely on black and white written communication, blueprints, interpersonal verbal communication skills, creativity, and exercise. Additionally, preferred jobs for the color blind often allow for technological assistance to determine color in a low-pressure situation, where accuracy and speed are not a part of the equation.

For instance, a friend of mine works a desk job that involves charting and graphing. Despite his color blindness, he thrives due to free, built-in technology and applications that assist him in color differentiation. His application allows him to determine color with a simple scroll of the mouse. He puts his cursor over the unidentified color, and the color name pops up!

Tip#64: Market your color blindness as an asset.

In many careers, color blindness is an advantage. My friend said his color deficiency aids his office work. In an effort to benefit all readers, he uses his color blindness to create graphs and charts that color blind people can easily read and process. He avoids red-green color schemes. Of course, his natural eye is the perfect gage for these color blind friendly charts. Without his handicap, his employers would have to rely on secondary resources and research instead of a primary source.

Color blindness primarily benefits my areas of expertise. As an English teacher, musician, and writer, I encounter very few color-complicated situations. Working primarily with black and white composition paper, staff paper, or computer screen, only descriptions of color pose a problem in my areas of expertise.

In fact, precision in color vocabulary enhances my color understanding. I am much more likely to write violet than purple or garnet than red. Sometimes the verbosity needed to describe a scene or character enhances a story much more than a few color words. Wouldn't you rather hear about the sun reflecting on the placid lake like a piece of glass that had fallen from heaven, than that the lake was still and blue! Color places limitations on our understanding sometimes and several jobs can benefit from your unique perspective as a color blind employee.

Least Likely Careers

While a color blind person can succeed in any career, it is important to understand which careers historically pose a problem for the color blind. In such careers, a color mishap could create a dangerous situation or an incorrect product. Let us delve in.

Tip#65: Avoid careers that pose a color safety or health concern

If color blindness interferes with safety or health concerns of your profession, either find another career or access the correct tools. Pilots and other transportation-related jobs historically have proven unsafe for color blind applicants because color determination in a quick time frame is necessary. Train cars have been derailed and planes crashed, costing lives, due to color blindness. If you have a "calling" to one of these careers, please divulge your color blind handicap and work with your boss to seek corrective equipment. Count the cost before pursuing such a career. It will be much harder to defect after investing your time, money, and energy into a career that ultimately will not be a good match. Plus, your employer may spring a color blind test on you last minute. Do not attempt to memorize the answers, as this is not only dangerous, but the tester can quiz you backwards or in any order he or she prefers.

Some types of engineering, like electrical, require color blind tests. Employers may not offer the color blind test until after the applicant has accepted the job, but they will cancel the contract immediately if color poses a safety concern. Before pursing an education or career that requires color determination, ask about color blindness as a prerequisite. While electrical engineering does not have an international prerequisite, you may find that an individual company, or several of them, will reject your application. While cheating on the color blind test tempts applicants, I strongly advise against it. Watch a few safety videos on arch flashes or other electrical explosions, and you will realize the potential for material and human loss.

While several doctors report color blindness, thoughtfulness is required from the applicant. For instance, if your color deficiency interferes with determining if a patient has a certain disease, such as the yellow in jaundice, you may need to ask for assistance on a regular basis. Ascertain that such help is available and that you feel comfortable seeking assistance regularly. As a mom, I constantly consult the doctor to help me determine the color of a rash or bruise, and I expected that the professional could provide such assistance. Doctors in a high-paced, dangerous situation, such as the emergency room or wartime situation, must be able to make quick color decisions. First responders, such as firefighters and policeman, demand accurate color vision as well. It is literally a matter of life or death.

Tip#66: Other jobs may pose several color-related concerns that are not safety or health issues.

Some careers rely on color-accurate eyes to determine a precise final product. For instance, paint mixers need to blend a variety of color hues to create a precise match. We all know that the mis-tinted gallons sell for a fraction of the regular price. With the diversity of precise colors available today, a color blind person could easily fill a shelf with mis-tinted paints and ultimately cost their company a lot of money (and maybe themselves, their job). It is wise not to commit to a job you know you cannot perform. But, perhaps, there is technology or another method to circumvent this conundrum. A life-long Crayola employee recently retired and disclosed his color blindness. His handicap never affected his lengthy career as a crayon maker.

Other jobs involve large merchandise orders, such as matching jerseys. If your job requires ordering color-precise items in bulk, be extra vigilant. While an occasional wrong order might get a blind eye, reoccurring incorrect large purchase orders will cost a company beaucoup bucks and might cost you your job. Once again, it is wise to not get in over your head.

Do Not Dismiss - Standing Out in Your Profession

Several color blind people have been so successful in their careers that they have reached celebrity status. For instance, Bill Clinton became president. Yes, the

United States has not had a woman president, but we have had a color blind president! Other political figures include Marco Rubio, Bob Dole, and Prince William Windsor. Mark Zuckerberg, founder and owner of Facebook, revealed that he is colorblind and chose the bright blue color for his franchise because it is the easiest to see. In the arts, Howie Mendel, Paul Newman, Bing Crosby, Fred Rogers, Christopher Nolan, Mark Twain and Meatloaf all mix up their colors. The list goes on and on, proving that color blind people can accomplish anything!

On a more personal note, while mingling at a meet and greet with a retired art teacher who continues to create art for children's books, I mentioned my color blindness and attempted to inquire about his experience with color blind students. Much to my dismay, he interrupted me to exclaim, "I am color blind!" Sacre Bleu (or purple)! How amazing!

My new best friend proceeded with his life story as a color blind person. He did not discover his handicap until he was in college art class. Able to sense which colors fit together, but unable to identify them, he would use phrases like, "tone it down," instead or "use lavender instead of violet." Additionally, his color blindness prevented him from serving in the air force but did not thwart his honorable service in the army ROTC.

The rest is history. Retired as a beloved art teacher, he continues to sculpt, paint, and illustrate with beautiful interpretation and symbolism. His artwork conveys something much more profound than a color wheel, because true art is from the heart.

Tip#67: Do not let color blindness stand between you and your dream. If an art teacher can be color blind then you can reach your goal, too!

Consider interior design, which is highly color sensitive. If you are working within a familiar color scheme, focus on the characteristics that make your style unique. Joanna Ganes in her Magnolia Home magazine focuses on much more than color. She highlights plants, texture, placement, layout, time periods, and much more. If a leading designer is not preoccupied with color, you do not have to be either. Plus, you have the superior eye to notice the extra elements without being distracted by color. You may even discover a color combination others were too afraid to try.

Tip#68: When a career does not pan out due to color blindness, pursue it as a hobby.

When my husband and I remodeled our house, I answered the call of interior decorator. I do not think I could make the cut in the professional interior design world, but my own castle only begs my own approval (and maybe my inmates, a.k.a family). I became hyper aware of my color blindness. Drawing upon Sherwin Williams' color match cards and salespeople's tips, I gleaned a few ideas. But a nagging feeling told me to follow my gut. And I did...

With dark blue, bright but mild yellows, and grays throughout my kitchen remodel, I have a unique, welcoming feel. Guests welcome the colors in my house and invite a break from the typical tans or blues. In fact, when I researched my color schemes during a continued renovation, I found all my senses

68

were correct. The dark blue mellowed out the yellow with its contrasting color. The gray provided a perfect neutral that would downplay the brightness of the other colors. Other tricks I played with patterns, plants, and spacing, also aligned with the professional tips! Although a career change is not on the horizon, I learned a new skill and boosted my color blind self-esteem.

Tip#69: Everyone has limitations, some more inhibiting than color blindness.

Reading this entire book may give you the impression that the color blind population deserves pity for the plethora of challenges and restrictions we face. However, much more severe conditions exist. Let us put our handicap in perspective for a moment. Terminal illnesses, congenital diseases, mental and physical handicaps, poverty, and abuse affect the global population at rampant rates. While these issues can affect color blind people, we need not forget to count our blessings and remember that our weaknesses should unite, not divide, us from others.

Chapter Review:

Color blind people can pursue any career they set their hearts and mind toward, but prudence should be exercised. Research the likelihood of hire for a color blind person in your field of study before you are too invested. Remember that putting others in peril by cheating on a color blind test is not conscionable. Consider other ways to pursue an area of interest, such as switching from electrical to civil engineering. Perhaps write, market, or educate on a field of interest in which your handicap prevents safe performance. In fact, your unique perspective may provide helpful insight that otherwise would go untapped. Lastly, remember that you can always practice your passion as a hobby and that you are not in this alone.

Chapter 6: Can Color Blindness Enhance My Extracurricular Activities?

Hobbies provide a venue to practice new skills and interests both color-related and not. Without extracurricular activities, life would be rather gray. Do not let your color limitations stand in the way of your passions. Instead, bring your color blind bent to play at sports, music, or whatever endeavor you pursue in order to lend perspective. Nonetheless, read on to discover some tips for navigating new interests with a color blind eye.

The Great Outdoors

Beautiful to touch, see, smell, taste, and feel, the great outdoors appeal to every sense! Plus, many of our favorite activities take place outside, on a sports field, in a garden, or even on a trail. So how does the color blind population enjoy these hobbies while managing their limitations? This hardy breed does quite well. With a little laughter, ingenuity, and humility, color blind individuals find many outdoor hobbies rewarding.

Dominating in Sports

Perfect for us color bind folk, sports require very little color discrepancy. Relying on speed, agility, dexterity, strategy, fitness, and other skill sets, color blind people can dominate in sports without heavily factoring in their disability. Even so, a few quick tips can help with certain areas of trial.

Tip#70: Memorize teammates and opponents by distinctive features.

Most recreational, school, or other sports team organizations use colored jerseys to identify teams. Although almost always distinguishable, some team colors may appear similar to even the slightest of color blind players. For instance, a neon green jersey may appear bright yellow to a color deficient player. Therefore, always memorize teammates starting on the first practice. Also note distinctive features, like ponytails, glasses, colors of footwear or any other characteristic that may aid quick recognition mid-game. Noting these features on the opposing team can help with quick play as well. Employ this trick most effectively in games like soccer and basketball, where teams intermix on the playing surface.

While I have never had difficulty determining teammates or opponents during game play, I have often struggled to communicate on what color team friends played. Although I memorized my team's color, I never exerted the energy to identify the colors of every other team. Therefore, reading color-coded brackets posed a problem, and I typically referred to team names, player numbers, or other factors to communicate about a league.

Tip#71: Do not rule out leadership positions.

Mentioned in chapter five, my color blind office friend who creates charts and graphs runs a non-profit youth baseball league. Using his collegiate baseball skills and other talents, he manages a plethora of teams who encourage youth to play with precision and sportsmanship. Like any association, however, his duties include purchasing colored merchandise.

Tip#72: Always approve color-related sports association purchases with a color-accurate person.

The youth baseball director ordered a banner for his youth baseball association. Upon arrival via mail, he asked his wife and children what color it was. Expecting navy blue, he was surprised when his family responded with a resounding "purple." Before ordering a replacement, he ascertained the color with his family. While this led to some lighthearted laughter for my friends, had the order included hundreds of jerseys, it may not have been such a laughing matter. Always double check your color-related purchase, especially large orders, with a color-accurate friend.

Tip#73: Color blind professional sports players and fans unite!

Leaving sports to the professionals? No problem. Or is there? Color deficient fans and professional players alike have reported color deficiency issues and have brought awareness to their handicap more heavily in the past decade. The opening game to the Summer 2018 Men's World Cup confused color blind viewers who could not distinguish between the red and green jerseys of Russia and Saudia Arabia teams respectively. Color blind viewers were left questioning who passed, threw, or scored during the game. In the same vein, professional athletes have reported difficulty viewing game balls, such as an orange golf or field hockey ball against green grass or the pink substitutionary ball used in cricket night games. Such difficulty imposes a huge disadvantage because time and precision are of essence in these games. Still, professional sports have barely given color blindness a head nod, and perhaps because we hold our own. To increase awareness, nonetheless, speak out on social media, local sports teams, or any opportunity that rolls your way.

Sports provide a healthy and fun outlet for color blind individuals without presenting serious color-related challenges. Whether on the field, couch, or in the locker room, color blind athletes contribute to the games we all know and love. Through strategies such as memorization, teamwork, and advocacy, color blind athletes will continue to dominate in sports.

Gardening

From the therapeutic dirt digging to the rewarding fresh vegetables and bouquets, gardening offers an array of payoffs. With recent raw food trends and micro-farming on the rise, gardening tips run aplenty, but how do the color blind gardeners navigate the color-related aspects of the trade?

Tip#74: Garden with a color-accurate partner.

From discerning composite rich soil to picking ripe vegetables, the color blind gardener can glean insights from color-accurate partners. Initially spearheading our garden, my husband has passed on his wisdom, and sometimes the baton, to me, his color blind wife. The years of shadowing him and gleaning gardening knowhow proved priceless this gardening season, as I planted, weeded, and harvested much of the crop alone. Before you attempt gardening alone, consider embracing the role of apprentice.

Tip#75: Touch the soil to determine its health and readiness for planting.

While sight can play a large role in assessing soil readiness for planting, touching the soil, especially for the color blind, provides just as much feedback. While the color-accurate may glance at soil for a light brown or dark brown appearance, the color blind may find this assessment difficult.

To use the touch test, first remember that different types of vegetables and flowers need different types of soil, so research the plant and its needs before planting. Most plants, however, need a darker, wetter, workable soil that is easy to turn with the hands and allows for roots to take and soak up rainwater. Some plants, however, require drier or firmer soil depending on their native growing conditions or other factors. For instance, carrots need a looser soil to allow their long noses to grow deep and wide within the ground. Assess your soil through touch, looking for a sandy-like texture. If the texture is incorrect, mix in sand. If your color blindness interferes with assessing the health of soil, use touch to assess if it is wet, dry, loose, or firm.

Tip#76: Memorize the shapes and stages of new plant growth, along with the appearances of weeds and other noxious items.

With optimum soil and gardening conditions, your plants will sprout within the indicated timeframe. Avoid the rookie and color blind mistake of uprooting new, bright green growth. Color-accurate gardeners will spot the bright color of new growth, but we may not be able to rely on our color senses to guide us correctly. The various shades of green within a garden are endless, so memorizing the shapes of a sprout, along with the noxious weeds thriving alongside, will prevent accidental uprooting. This is especially important if your crop requires thinning, such as pulling carrot sapling once they are an inch tall to allow roots room to develop full fruits.

Tip#77: Planting in a pattern wards off accidental uprooting.

In addition to memorizing plants shapes and sizes, along with stages of growth, planting in a pattern will prevent accidental uprooting. Whether you are planting in a raised bed or directly in the ground, organizing your crops in straight rows will help prevent accidental uprooting. Anything growing outside the row requires weeding; whereas outlier can be pulled. Sometimes animals or wind will scatter or disorganize your crop, but typically the pattern will stand. Organization circumvents color determination.

Tip#78: Little bugs, withering leaves, dried stems – blight attacks when least expected.

These gardening diseases steal our fruits and veggies by spreading from plant to plant and executing garden genocide. While my husband spots the devilish doom immediately, sometimes I cannot see the blight in plain sight. The dotted leaves appear uniform to me or the darkening rim does not register with my eyes. When my husband is unusually busy with work during the summer, sometimes blight can take hold before my eyes register it. Catching blight late can result in the loss of the plant and its yield. Studying specific blights to which your plants are prone, can help you spot the blight sooner. For instance, tomatoes and other fruits in their family experience an early and late blight, the former showcasing spots and the latter forming a brown rim around leaves. Knowing when to look and how each blight manifests, helps the color blind identify these potentially deadly plant diseases.

Tip#79: Use seed packets and other gardening resources to create a harvesting calendar.

While color-accurate gardeners rely on sight to determine ripeness and readiness for harvesting, color blind individuals need additional guidelines. Although tomatoes grow in a variety of colors, most commonly, tomatoes are ready to harvest when they are red or almost red. Tomatoes can ripen off the vine; therefore, early picking is okay. In fact, some culinarians, or country bumpkins, prefer fried green tomatoes.

Nonetheless, tomato harvesting for a delectable, robust sauce or ketchup requires accurate picking. For the color blind harvester, distinguishing between green, orange, and red tomatoes may be problematic. If planted from seed, the packet should reveal how many days until harvest. Plants purchased at a nursery include informational tags that reveal the plants' name, germination period, harvest requirements, and more. If you misplace a tag or it contains sparse information, consult a gardener's encyclopedia or website. Marking a calendar with harvesting dates for each vegetable will avoid early or late picking.

Although your calendar will provide an accurate harvesting timeframe, environmental factors, such as rain and sunshine, weigh in as well. Within the appropriate time frame, check your vegetables by sight and other senses. For fruit like tomatoes, touch the skin to judge ripeness. If the tomato looks red to you, pierces easily, and has a slight give to it flesh when pressured, pick it. Remember, picking vegetables too early is not a cardinal sin. Recipes exist for all stages of ripeness; plus, unripe veggies can always feed the chickens or benefit the compost.

I could fill a book with my color-related gardening mistakes, but a paragraph will have to suffice. First, I have allowed my kids to eat half bushels of unripe tomatoes that appeared red but were orange in reality. A pack of toilet paper later, my children and I had learned our lesson the hard way. Strained orange tomato juice served as the base for sour soups and sauces that were edible but not relished. Similar stories ensued with strawberries, whose green/red harvesting spectrum pose comparable concerns as tomatoes. Overripe, desiccated green beans and underripe, tooth-breaking green peppers have adorned my dinner table. Through trial and error, attention to non-color harvesting details, and a little grace, I have managed to heavily outweigh my farm-to-table flub ups with farm fresh, scrumptious meals.

Hiking

Hiking tops the charts as a favorite outdoor pastime due to its various health benefits and multiple degrees of commitment. Fresh air, stunning views, a lazy stroll, or a brisk walk appeal to a myriad of people, including the color blind. We, however, may enjoy the musky fragrance of crinkly leaves beneath our boots more than their colorful display in the fall. Apart from the sensory experiences that hiking presents, more notable obstacles may cross the color blind hiker's path.

Tip#80: Be alert for camouflage trail markings!

Most of my hikes begin without preparation when a whim hits for trekking the great outdoors. Typically, I'll enter a local or state park and follow their natural paths with rocky and root-laden paths. Often sparsely maintained, theses trails often include overgrown areas where the walkway becomes unclear. At such junctions, hikers rely on spray-painted markings on trees that disclose the correct direction. Unless, of course, the spray paint is a streak of green, brown, or red atop brown bark. While the color-accurate hiker simply follows the tree markings, the color blind hiker is left to guesswork. I have made some trails of my own when the path became unclear, and fortunately, I have never ended up over a cliff or in a lake. Nonetheless, it is wise to attempt to identify the tree markings as soon as possible, bring a hiking buddy, or stick to well-known trails.

Tip#81: Hot hiking brings sunburn!

While the idea of hiking calls to mind shady trails and overhead canopies, sometimes hiking and other outdoor activities involve lots of sun exposure. An unplanned hike may include miles of sunny steps that leave you red, especially if you cannot see pink well. I can recall many hikes, beach vacations, days at the pool, and other sun-filled endeavors that ended with blisters and aloe lotion.

Although color-accurate friends can see sunburn forming, starting with a light pink and increasing in intensity, we may only be able to spot the burn once it is red and painful. Sometimes I never see the sunburn but feel its intensity in the shower as water burns like acid rain. The best defense against sunburn for the color blind is similar to typical sun care suggestions. Wear sunscreen, hats, SPF clothing, and follow other basic sun exposure guidelines. I recently purchased Columbia Sportwear SPF shirts and shorts for a hiking trip and can report in hindsight that I did not experience any sunburn and felt comfortable hiking the entire time. And if someone says your shoulders or nose look pink, take a hint and reapply.

The Liberal Arts

Foundational for our enjoyment of life, the liberal arts draw upon our deeper sense of self, one that transcends the superficialities of sight. Engaging our minds, hearts, and sundry senses, the liberal arts fling wide open the door for the color blind. This chapter will highlight how our color blindness can help create an exceptional experience and expression of the liberal arts for both personal satisfaction and sharing purposes.

Tip#82: Use your superpowers (aka: other senses).

In a world that grabs our attention through our eyes, let us talk about engaging our other senses. Like a blind person may have an enhanced sense of smell or hearing, so you might have an enhanced sense. Consider the senses you have substituted for sight in various situations. Does taste, alone, tell you when dinner is done? Do you buy clothing based on how it feels? Or perhaps you might just find more enjoyment in another sensual experience. For instance, do you love to listen to music? It comes from the heart, as the old country song goes. With our eyes closed, it provides color and beauty to our world.

Music

Perhaps you need an outlet for your passion and visual arts has fallen flat for you. Consider expressing your passion through sound rather than sight. Although sound is color blind, it expresses, evokes, and captures emotion just as gloriously. In fact, music is a color in itself. Paint me some Mozart or Handle. Add a new hue with some Billy Joel or Lynyrd Skynyrd. With some training, you can create your own masterpiece with minimal color blind obstacles.

Tip#83: Music is color blind like us.

Unless you are studying child's lesson series, color does not conflict with music. Learning to read music is much like learning to read books or solve math problems in that it bypasses color confusion. You bring the color to the music through your passion.

Tip#84: Color your world with music!

Just like sunshine yellow, lifts our spirits, so does the right song at the right time. The color blind may not be able to see the sunshine yellow in its brightest state, but we can play or sing a song that evokes that same feeling. In fact, a friend's husband plays the guitar by ear. She asked him what he sees when his eyes are closed and he is jamming. He described it as all the colors of the rainbow floating around. What a beautiful description for the color-accurate and color blind alike. Nonetheless, while this description sounds lovely to me, I cannot relate. My friend asked if this was my experience with music, and I had a resounding "no." When I play the piano, I see the notes. Even with my eyes closed, I have never seen color. Rather I feel raw emotion, like I am telling the most poignant narrative without any words. Colors never entered my mind, but the same tangible beauty did!

Engage your inner beauty and color your world through music. With a variety of instruments, genres, and much more, music can provide the outlet you need for genuine self-expression.

Cooking

I love to cook. At one point in young motherhood, I cooked every meal, every day. I even grew my own food and made my own spaghetti sauce. Add to that, fresh eggs, and you get the idea that I am a foodie. But being color blind and cooking present some challenges, both obvious and hidden.

Tip#85: Using your multiple senses will enhance your cooking!

Ladies and gentlemen, we are blessed not to rely on our sense of sight when it comes to cooking. For the regular cook, it is simply easier to *see* when something is finished cooking but for the true chef, the other senses must be engaged. As color blind cooks, we have a natural advantage because we are forced to use our other senses. Let us see how this benefits us!

Tip#86: Refining your sense of taste will elevate your cooking!

Woe to the chef who cannot taste his own sauce! Try, try, try everything. You tongue makes a much better judge than your eye, which can deceive even the color-accurate. A roux might look golden and nutty, but upon taste, you may discover it needs a longer cook time. Taste, taste, taste. This is no time to trust your eye. It is, however, a perfect time to refine your palette.

My family and I love to play "guess that food." With the children, we will eat all sorts of food, even odd combinations, with our eyes closed. This is an excellent, and fun, way to train your palette and to make new flavor discoveries.

More useful, however, is memorizing herbs by their taste and smell. Close your eyes and ask a team player to hold an herb under your nose. After wafting the herb, have the teammate deposit a mite in your hand. After tasting, guess the herb. Once you have played the game multiple times, you will have memorized several herbs by taste and smell. Now you can season your cooking like a professional and without relying on your sense of sight. With a little work and adaptation, you could apply this game to whatever cooking items cause your eye the most problems.

Tip#87: Using your finger and other "tools"

Use a meat thermometer. Whenever possible, gauge when something is finished by temperature. Any recipe worth its salt (pun intended), will include an internal temperature and directions on where to insert the tool. This is especially important with meats that dry out easily like porkchops. While the color-accurate will simply glance to ascertain the correct color, we may not be able to distinguish the various shades of pink to brown.

Resist the temptation to halve a piece of meat and check for color. In addition to our obvious impairment, cutting into a piece of meat to check for readiness is not ideal anyhow because it interrupts the cooking process. If you do not own or desire to purchase a meat thermometer, use the touch test. If the steak has a lot of give, like the padding on your middle finger, it is closer to rare. If the steak is firmer, like your index finger's padding, it is closer to medium. A very tough steak to the touch is done or well-done.

Apply the touch test to other food items. If you cannot determine if a cake looks golden and cooked through, touch it slightly for bounce back. Depending on your recipe and if you have used the toothpick test yet, you may need to let the cake cool a bit before trying this. It should bounce back if it is done.

Tip#88: Sense of smell

Trust your nose. After baking a few goodies, you'll know when the batter goldens by its fragrant smell. If your house starts to smell like a candle was blown out recently, your food is overdone. Apply the nose test to meats, vegetables, and other oven roasted items. Typically, they will smell sweet when done and quickly transition to a burnt scent. To bypass mistakes made with the eye, train your nose to pick up on these fragrances quickly. Otherwise, you may end up relying on the smoke detector!

Tip#89: Using your eye

Sometimes stovetop meals interfere with the nose test. While a fresh chicken or meat might exude an aromatic smell while sautéing in a pan, most times it is too tempting to rely on your eye. Just remember that a browned meat or cooked chicken will no longer look pink. Do not look for brown or any other distinctive color; look for "no longer pink."

Sometimes your meal will go awry due to your color blindness; remember that you are in control. If you see black/burnt meat, remove your dish immediately from the heat and evaluate. You probably overcooked it. Heavy sauce, both red or white, can help disguise this rookie mistake and recover your meal.

Use your eye for fun! Just like with interior design or clothing trends, incorporating color into your cooking is totally in your wheelhouse. You do not have to skip this approach because of your deficit. Mix various colors of carrots or potatoes together for a unified taste with an alluring presentation. Mix fruits for an eye-catching side dish.

Tip#90: Relying on the pros and foodie trends

From the country kitchen to the streets of Paris, any style of cooking benefits from expert advice. In fact, the color blind cook can sidestep several challenges by following the advice of Ree Drummond or Julia Child. Exact measurements, techniques, and other pointers quickly transfer expert tips to any cook and especially the uncertain color blind cook.

I am mildly obsessed with the pioneer woman and have read an autobiography on Julia Child. Their life stories provide further evidence that cooking is an experiment. Mistakes are welcome. Even Disney movies like "Ratatouille" assert, "Anyone can cook." That includes us!

The crock pot and similar devices have made a significant impact on modern cooking, mostly due to their convenience in our busy, modern society. However, the crock pot benefits the colorblind because it circumvents several obstacles color blind cooks face. For instance, the crock pot typically runs on a timer, and food is thoroughly cooked without under or overcooking due to a liquid bath or other ingredients present in the pot. Still, use your nose and other senses to catch crock pot pitfalls (like a faulty crock pot).

Tip#91: Look for other reasonable causes for your kitchen mishaps.

Whatever happens in the kitchen, stays in the kitchen. Do not let a mishap due to color blindness deter you from further ventures. Even color accurate home chefs ruin a meal now and again. I went through a stage of life where grilling a homemade hamburger proved a herculean feat. Upon biting into his burger, my husband would politely recoil. Detecting undercooked meat, I immediately assumed my color blindness had interfered with my cooking. Sometimes the children ate their burger a bit raw, and no one got sick. However, once we purchased a new grill, my hamburgers significantly improved. Low and behold, the grill, not my color deficiency, undercooked my burgers (or so I concluded). Before assuming the problem is you, look at other reasonable causes.

Do not deprive your sense of taste because your sense of sight is lacking. Rather, indulge your senses by applying them to your cooking. With the right tools, books, and your natural instincts, you can cook like a pro. So, go ahead and host Thanksgiving dinner, the neighborhood block party, or a romantic meal for your lover. You have got this!

Unique Take on Color-Related Activities

Color is in the eye of the beholder. One person calls a turquoise shirt green, while another calls it blue. While we obviously have blind spots in our color spectrum, we also have opinions and preference on color that are unrelated to our handicap. Let your unique color views shine through on the professional stage and in your own home.

Tip#92: When involved in a color-related activity, redefine yourself as color deficient.

Due to a lack of education about color blindness, most people do not know much about our handicap. People will assume that you either cannot see color or that one or more colors is missing completely. While this may be true for some of us, most of us only confuse a few shades of one or two colors. Therefore, it is imperative that you set the record straight. No one else is going to do it for you! Let your cohorts know that you can see almost every color perfectly. As annoying as it is, let them test you for color accuracy. Have fun with the extra attention and debunking some myths about our "condition." Once your associates know that you can see color well, they will stop excluding you from color-related activities and discussions. Plus, they will know accurately about your weakness, so they can help you when it is necessary.

Tip#93: Your house is your kingdom!

As far as your house is concerned, you can decide how to decorate it; yes, including color! Do not be intimidated. Paint stores are more than accommodating to the color blind. If you want good service, chose a store that specializes exclusively in paint, like Sherwin Williams. Their everyday workers will help you pick out colors, mix and match, and much more. Trust me, I live within a mile of one. If you want to seek extra advice, they offer in-home consultants to evaluate your color schemes and help design your personalized palate. This service is free if you purchase your paint at their store.

Perhaps you want to "do it yourself." This is more my style! Almost all paint cards offer accompanying colors. For instance, I painted my living room green. I wanted multiple shades of green that I could mix with gold and brown for a clean, earthy, vintage look. With such vision in mind, I selected the color cucumber water. It is a very light green that almost appears tan to my eye. However, I know it is green because the color cards are organized so meticulously by color and shade. As if that is not enough, the back of the card reports a color reflectivity number. This number explains how much light will reflect off the selected color. Additionally, the card includes complementary colors. I chose a pistachio green for my baseboard and trim. The card noted that cream colors match as well, so I did not even need to paint my cream ceiling. I bounced these ideas off of the Sherwin Williams consultant and my artsy mother-in-law, and the rest is history. My living room is so unique, relaxing, and colorful.

Setting the record straight about your color deficiency and practicing your color choices in the comfort of your home provides instant validation for your color abilities. Do not box yourself out of the fun color-related activities in life because of what you or others think about your color capabilities. Practice makes perfect, and with a little ingenuity, you can make satisfying color choices!

From outdoor to indoor activities and everything in-between, the color blind can contribute and enjoy any hobby that ignites their passion. Overcoming color-related obstacles with simple knowhow frees us up to let our talents shine as we serve our families, express ourselves, and bring a little color to our lives.

Chapter 7: How Can I Live My Best Life With Color Blindness

Being Positive

Not to sound trite, but being positive is a solution in itself. Sometimes a plan to handle a unique color blind problem is right around the corner, but we have to travel to it or wait for it to travel to us. While we are in a state of uncertainty or embarrassment, staying positive keeps ourselves and our relationships in good working order. Let us peek at a few ways to stay positive when your color blindness has you down.

Tip#94: A good sense of humor covers a multitude of errors.

Whether your clothes do not match or you undercooked the chicken again, laughing at yourself is the quickest way to relieve the tension. We all know the platitudes- laugh at yourself before anyone else can. But really, the mark of ownership with color blindness rings out in a cackle. I have served moldy bread, eaten unripe bananas, and brought an uncharged camera to a party (those darn color -coded battery life strips), but laughed it off because it wasn't my fault – we were born this way.

Tip#95: Never stop looking for resolutions.

Ownership of your handicap does not rule out your right to find corrective measures. Just a quick Google search will reveal a multitude of articles and videos tooting EnChorma glasses that can enhance a color blind person's vision. Although I haven't personally tried these gizmos, I give my blessing to anyone who desires to give it a whirl. At only around $269 for child glasses and $349 for an adult pair, this affordable accessory may provide a temporary solution for your color blindness. I am happy with how green my grass is, but if your acute color blindness bothers you, maybe the grass *will* be greener with EnChroma!

Tip#96: Do not blame others.

Sometimes negative energy causes us to blame others for our problems. If your positive chi is running low, remember to refrain from blaming others. Perhaps your boss won't make proper accommodations for your color blindness or a teacher denies your need for assistance. Refrain from blaming others, and appeal to a higher power. Perhaps the Americans with Disabilities Act can plea for you at work or the Individuals with Disabilities Education Act for your needs at school. Find some allies and politely get the help you need. If the boulder won't move, walk around it. Perhaps a new job or school would benefit from your assets more than the unhelpful place you reside.

Staying positive about your condition will help you overcome your struggles in the best manner. Own your handicap with laughter, know your options for improvement, and affirm your rights in the public sphere. Let us set positivity as the precedence while we remain outspoken and honest about our color blindness and the need for education and understanding in the private and public sphere.

Being Humble

Humility gets a bad rap in our modern, global, competitive society. We continually self promote as we climb the corporate ladder. Even in our neighborhoods, schools, and churches, we jockey for the best position. While our competition increases our skills, it often overlooks the strength we can find in our weakness. As color blind people, let us take a look at how our handicap can strengthen our character.

Tip#97: Let your weakness increase your faith.

Living with color blindness has increased my faith. From a young age, I have had to rely on other people to inform me of colors. Even when my senses told me the other person was wrong, I had to trust him or her. This happened with not only friends, but with my family member, whom may suffer from color blindness as well.

Anyhow, trusting in color has been like trusting in my religious faith. My belief system chooses to love every time, encouraging compassion, forgiveness, and other loving qualities even when they seem illogical. The most illogical action for a human is to put others first; we are wired to look out for number one. But the truth is that my self-interest is not always what is most important. Sometimes the needs of family members, friends, or the community are more important than our own agenda and benefit us the most in the long run. Even when it seems illogical, my faith asserts that the truest color in relationships is love and altruism. Through color blindness, I have learned that the truth is not always apparent at first sight.

One of my favorite religious writings reads, "We live by faith, and not by sight."2 Corinthians 5:7. With color blindness, I literally do that every day. So, when I cannot see what my future holds, I remember there are a lot of things I cannot see, but life has been good to me!

Tip#98: Set your vanity aside.

With every accommodation and medical advancement available, we still cannot expect ourselves to preform like color-accurate people in color-related endeavors. All efforts implemented, we still might have a mismatching outfit or misread map. We must bravely laugh at our mistakes with those who understand.

My most embarrassing mishaps involve makeup because *they happened on my face*. It is hard for people to overlook something egregious on our faces. Consider Fred Savage's moley moley moley in Austin Powers. In polite society, however, social mores restrict such outlandish outburst, and while saving face, we are left to wonder if we made a huge color mistake.

At my church's county-wide Bible study, I sat amongst a multi-generational group of polite Christian women. Usually quite gregarious, several of them eyed me with suspicion or concern – I couldn't quite make it out until later that day. Upon returning home, I caught a glimpse of myself in the now well-lit mirror. To my dismay, my lips were outlined in bright orange lipstick! The lovely ladies had failed to inform me of my mishap. Not knowing that I was color blind, perhaps they thought I intended to treat myself to a Halloween makeover. In unabashed, unnerved laughter, I tossed the orange lipstick in the can.

Around the same time period, when I was starting to care for my looks again after birthing three babies in quick succession, I dabbed on a new rose-colored blush. Blending in with my pale skin, I brushed on some more and then some more, until I could see the pale color. Feeling pretty and dressed quite nicely because it was Christmas Eve, I confidently stopped into the barber shop with my two young sons. With the jingle of the entry bell, everyone glanced our way when my family entered. When they kept lingering, I felt beautiful. Until the admiration rapidly became stares or furtive glances. Immediately, and with no recourse, I realized my faux pas and sat calmly with my children in the waiting area. Although no one breathed a disparaging word, my cheeks were "bright pink."

It is what we do with our weaknesses that really inform who we are. Since ours is relatively nonrestrictive, but definitely limiting, let us show each other and the world how we live humbly with our handicap. Maybe we'll inspire someone whose struggle is weighing them down.

Tip#99: Ask for more time or help to complete something.

Sometimes completing a task may take us more time or more accommodations, but really our disability must be respected. We should not be marginalized in the workplace due to the Americans with Disabilities Act, and we must assume respect at home. For instance, my husband politely assisted me in checking our pool's pH level this summer and guided me in comparing the chemical strip to the key. After his assistance, I realized that my color vision was strong enough for the task, which has little major repercussions, and did not need assistance in the future.

Tip#100: Color blindness should not be assumed as rudeness.

Thankfully, I did not need assistance in determining if I was pregnant or reading other female-related medical tests, but these are real possibilities. Ladies, if your husband cannot tell if the pregnancy test is positive or negative, do not get mad; inform him. Even in the most significant of moments, a color blind person cannot overcome his or her disability. Maybe your significant other cannot see the color drain from your face due to fear or the red rising to your cheeks due to embarrassment; be clear with them about your feelings. They are not ignoring your emotions; they cannot detect them by sight alone.

In the lifelong lesson of humility, we have a front row seat. We entered the classroom at birth when our color blindness had already been imprinted on our IEP for life. Regardless of how we handle our day-to-day affairs, our color blindness will promote humility if we live in truth and love. Let us pass the test of humility with flying colors.

Being Proud

"Why be a rock, when you really are a gem?" asks hip hop artist Lauryn Hill. Truly, it is our differences that make us stand out in this world. Pride in our uniqueness opens unusual doors of opportunity – like writing an eBook on color blindness.

Tip#101: A lighthearted and confident approach to your color blind story will help you respond to others' questions while acting as a role model to your children and others.

Since I have accepted this writing opportunity, friends and family have lavished me with attention. Friends, who never knew I had this handicap, politely asked questions reminiscent of my childhood days (is this blue or purple?). If you are not aware, this is the most annoying question for a color blind person; we do not know what color it is! However, I am able to respond, not react, in an adult manner now, as opposed to my younger days of rolling my eyes or ignoring the inquirer. While basic color blind questions may seem silly or bothersome to us, we need to remember that uninformed friends and family are lovingly and willingly trying to understand our plight. How excellent an opportunity to share our stories!

Also, some adults will respond with teasing (is it not funny how the kindergarten methods carry into adulthood?). Keep your standards and remember to respond maturely. As an adult, we can welcome kindhearted jesting with our own jibes and smiles or even explanations when necessary.

My father-in-law's relentless teasing provides the fodder for this chapter. He and my mother-in-law dinned with my husband, myself, and my parents one warm summer evening. Quite smitten with my newfound book gig to write about color blindness, he worked it into every comment. When I read something incorrectly, my color blindness was to blame. When I burned the food, he quipped that my colorblindness struck again. Boy do I wish I could blame all my failures on color blindness! His levity was a welcomed and expected attention from a loved one – he means well, and it is an opportunity to make light of what can sometimes be a difficult drawback.

Such lightheartedness helps your children as well. Whether your child has color blindness or not, he or she will certainly experience difficulties in life. Your child will need guidance and discussion, but as the old mantra goes – actions speak louder than words. As role models to our own children or those we encounter in day-to-day life, let us laugh and problem solve when color conundrums occur. I am constantly consulting my children on color-related matters. I ask my fashion-conscious and color-accurate son if his sibling's outfits match, sometimes even if mommy's outfit is color-coordinated. When a child is returned home by the school nurse due to pink eye, I shrug and consult the doctor. Despite my child's or my frustration, I let them know that I could not see the pink in their eyes, and everything will still be okay. Through our mishaps, we teach our children to admit their weaknesses and accept help.

A-Z Handbook

Always take your colorblindness into account. If you are struggling with something or someone, consider the possibility that your color blindness is interfering. For instance, you may not be able to distinguish a green belt from a brown or red belt in karate class. When you are not able to respond correctly, inform your instructor. Next, take the time to learn which students are of what rank and constantly update. Although the world should factor in our handicap, most of the time the hard work will fall on us.

Be honest about your disability. Hiding your disability could be unsafe, and stealth will most likely set a trap for yourself, not others. If your handicap is known, it will be easier to ask for help when color-related issues arise. Plus, you'll keep yourself out of unsafe positions.

Consult professionals for assistance with public affairs. When planning a large gathering or attending a gala, ask a party planner or fashion designer for help with color-coordination. You do not have to go it alone.

Dress for success by discovering your personal style in a color-friendly way. Shop in-store or online using my tips in chapter four. Drop your drab wardrobe, and don a look that screams confidence, style, and color (in whatever degree you desire).

Explain your child's condition to the authority figures in his or her life. Ascertain that teachers, coaches, grandparents, and step-parents understand the complications facing your color blind child. Use terms and scenarios that your audience can understand. Perhaps bring along a demonstration, such as a color by number, so individuals can witness the handicap firsthand. Sometimes seeing is believing ☺.

Find a support group. Connect with others who share your disability. While this won't enhance your color vision, walking alongside similar people allows for commiserating and correction. Keep abreast new developments in law and corrective wares, as you discuss your color conundrums with others. When life changes occur, such as moving to a new community for college or work, a support group can help with education about how to navigate the new locale as a color blind individual.

Genes discriminate when doling out color blindness. If we wore our genes like their homophonic cousin, each pant leg would need a defect for a female to wear them. Girls and women alike need a mutation on both of their sex(y) jeans to inherit color blindness. Males, however, would only need one ripped pant leg, or one gene to carry the mutation.

Handle color situations with finesse. Sometimes you have to walk the line with your color situation in order to maintain respect and authority. For instance, I never divulged my color blind handicap to my high school students when I taught 9th -12th grade English class. They would have quizzed me relentlessly and blamed every misnomer on my color deficiency. While that playfulness is fun with family and friends, it is a real deterrent to teaching, where you have to play God for a while. Typically, you can cover up your color blindness in a low stakes situation in order to remain authoritative, but do not risk this ruse as the underdog or in an unsafe situation. In those cases, decide who can and cannot handle your private information and how it will best behoove you.

Inheritance for color blindness comes through the woman. The woman passes color blindness onto her children through either having the mutation or being a carrier. Therefore, a son only needs her mutated gene or carrier gene to be color blind. This also leads us to believe that a color blind mom would have all color blind sons. Only one of my sons, however, is officially color blind. Maybe their disability will emerge later in life when color-accuracy is refined beyond primaries and simple colors. Or just maybe, science has some room research to do. My husband is color-accurate, and therefore my daughter is not color blind. She would need both mutations in order to inherit the disability. Check out my "G" tip for more on that.

Juxtaposition exposes color mishaps. If you have to make a quick color decision, find a color you know and hold the item in scrutiny next to it. Through comparison, you will be able to make your best guess. This does not work if you have monochromacy or black/white color blindness. Otherwise, this magic trick is just the abracadabra you need in a pinch.

Kids with color blindness require extra attention. While most kids want to ignore their color blindness, sometimes the parent, teacher, or other adult will need to intervene. Remember to grow with your child's needs. For example, little kids may need help getting dressed, school-aged kids may benefit from learning differentiation, preteens profit from fashion help, and teenagers require guidance as they discover how their handicap may impact their future choices. Walk beside your child, students, or other kids in your life by offering them a helping hand when color challenges prove a stumbling block.

Look to the future. While Enchroma glasses are the best current solution for color correction, scientific research continues for more permanent solutions. Researchers inquiring and experimenting with monkeys about single injection gene therapy report promising but perhaps risky results. Maybe the future will include safe, corrective surgery that will enable us to pursue our dreams in a safe and fair manner.

Mapping adaptations are available for the color blind. While I've never used a color blind adapted map, cartographers continually advance their mapping adaptations for people with monochromacy and an array of other color blind confusions. Search the internet, app store, AAA or other map carriers to find the right map for your next trip.

Never eat a food item in scrutiny. If you cannot discern whether the food in question is cooked, raw, moldy, or any other stage of inedibility, do not ingest it! Inedible foods do not discriminate, and you might pay the price. While my iron stomach has not betrayed me frequently, I can recall several mishaps with pink meat, green yogurt, and other unsavory items. Out of hunger or exhaustion, I am not sure, but I've told myself that these items did not look too far gone or perhaps they had "oxidized." So, with fair warning, heed my cautionary tales, and eschew dubious food items.

Orange might really be red. From the "orange" blinking light on a recording camera to the ubiquitous traffic lights, orange, as we color blind people see it, is often really red. Try memorizing what items are orange and which ones are red, but also expect that corrections will occur. When someone tells you that an "orange" item is really red, say thanks and add it to your color codex.

Peppers comes in multiple colors. I am just teasing. You obviously know this. But do not limit yourself to a boring culinary experience because you are unsure of certain colors. Red peppers are sweeter than green ones and may even present less digestion problems. Go ahead and ask the salesclerk which pepper is the red one. If this seems extremely embarrassing, explain your condition first. Most likely, the clerk will be enthralled and inquire about your handicap (presenting a perfect teaching opportunity) or he will show you where the desired vegetable resides. Happy shopping!

Quitting is not an option. Well, at least it should not be. While quitting a difficult job, hobby, or personal responsibility may provide some temporary relief, working through your color blind issue will produce the sort of character and knowhow you need in a color-seeing world. The world is not about to go color blind any day soon, so adapting to the reality of a color-accurate world is your best option. Talk to your boss, coach, spouse, or whoever can help remedy the problem. Bridging the color blind gap within your sphere of influence will set a precedence for other color blind comrades. Perhaps your efforts to acquire color blind modifications at your work will transfer to your protégée.

Respond instead of reacting to naysayers. If someone tries to deny your color blindness or treat you unfairly because of it, remain calm and look for reasonable solutions. This is particularly important for children, teens, and young adults who may feel under attack when others do not understand their limitations. As the world becomes more literate in color blindness, scientific advances are made, school districts incorporate it into IEPs, and other aspects of society adapt to our conditions, our handicap will join the ranks with other common limitations. Responding and representing our "people" well will soften society to making adaptions for us. If you are the parents, spouse, or otherwise representative for a color blind person, help guide your color blind friend by remaining calm and thoughtful when emotions are flying high. Together, we have got this!

Sense your way through things. Use all six senses: smell, touch, taste, sight, hearing, and thinking. Memorizing is the first line of attack for a color illiterate person but mundane and professional tasks often require real-time decisions. Use your nose to tell if food has spoiled or finished cooking. Touch steak to determine its doneness and taste your roux to decide if its color reflects the flavor your desire. Compare dubious colors to known ones to discover color compatibility in a pinch. Train your ear to indulge your musical senses and discover color-unrelated talents.

Total color blindness encompasses sight limited to black, white and the gray scale in-between. While this condition is extremely rare, it requires much more assistance and understanding from the community, family, friends, and neighbors who surround the sufferer. As the totally color blind person, seek out a color blind community in-person or online who can empathize with you. While your journey is unique, it is one of many arduous paths that each hiker in life must travail.

Undiscovered color blindness may or may not surface later in life. A later-in-life discovery may occur if color blindness is interfering with a job or daily tasks. Hopefully, this discovery does not interfere with a person's trajectory and results in little to no emotional, financial, or other means of strain or stress. Sometimes, a late discovery may cause embarrassment or actually interferences with life advancements, such as obtaining a job post-secondary education. In such cases, remember that accommodations are often available but safety and efficiency should be taken into consideration. To be cliché, when one door closes another one opens. Chin up! Maybe your disability can provide research assistance to your area of interest. Do not let your handicap define you but you define it!

Venture into uncharted territory with caution and confidence. Whether a new career, hiking trail, hobby, or other endeavor has caught your heart and mind, do not let your color blindness stand in the way. Rather, think through your new project and even conduct research if your safety may be at risk. Getting lost abroad, giving someone food poisoning, or panting your walls a heinous color may be avoidable with a little forethought.

Wear your rose-colored glasses (if pink is your color). Seriously though, remaining positive about any color challenges that surface will help you surmount them.

Your color blindness is not going away, unless you have found a safe, non-cumbersome alternative. In which case, shoot me an email.

X-ray vision is one of our superpowers. Well, not quite, but we can read x-rays because they generally appear in black, white, and grey. Which is great news if you want to be a radiologist. While there may be some color-related readings that could pose a problem, the majority of images will be readable for you.

Your friends and family are your best secret weapon. Worried about matching your clothing- text a friend. Need some tips with cooking- summon your spouse. Embarrassed about a color flub up- laugh with your neighbor. In a color crisis – ask your color savvy kid. Your friends and family can help you through almost any low-stakes color dilemma that comes your way.

Zany zeal. For real? Yes. Sometimes your color blindness will result in an outward display of craziness. If you do not feel like disclosing your color blindness of making excuses for who you are, just embrace it. Yes, we are a bit zany sometimes. Yes, we might appear to have a zeal for mismatching socks. Just live it up, and remember another z word (Zuckerberg). Perhaps Facebook would not have had the same appeal without its color blind founder picking a bright blue insignia. Find your inner Zuckerberg when zany zeal wants to wear you down.

About the Expert

With blue eyes and brown hair, your color blind author, Kimberly Springer, lives in the suburbs of Pittsburgh with her hazel-eyed husband, green-eyed oldest son, brown-eyed middle son, and blue-eyed little girl. Her tri-colored, purebred Basset Hound provides the perfect sidekick for calm days of writing, piano playing, and cooking. Despite her obvious inability to view every Fall color, Autumn remains Kim's favorite season due to the smoky air from fires, sundry warm beverages, scratchy hayrides, and flavorful Thanksgiving feasts.

On a more professional note, Kim hails from a diverse background of experience. You could describe her as quite the Philly Phanatic, born and raised just outside the city of brotherly love. Remaining loyal to her state, she attended The Pennsylvania State University in State College to study secondary education, specializing in English, communications, and journalism. As a Freshman, Kim wrote for the far-reaching Daily Collegian as a Senior reporter, followed by a stint as a Health and Wellness journalist. After serving as a community leader through school and church-appointed positions, Kim continued her travels west with an appointment to teach in the suburbs of Pittsburgh. There she met her husband of 10 years and graduated magna cum laude. Wielding both a teaching and marriage certificate, Kim entered the married and working world at a young age. As an educator, she has taught grades 7-12 in a variety of school-settings, including the acclaimed Lincoln Park Performing Arts Charter School in Midland, PA. Nowadays, she devotes her time to her family, home, church, piano students, and online writing. She believes in the power of everyday communication and education through online forums, community gatherings, and outreach activities to enhance the lives of all peoples. Be on the lookout for more items from Kim, as she hopes to continue to inform and entertain through the wonderful world of online literature.

HowExpert publishes quick 'how to' guides on all topics from A to Z by everyday experts. Visit HowExpert.com to learn more.

Recommended Resources

- <u>HowExpert.com</u> – Quick 'How To' Guides on All Topics by Everyday Experts.
- <u>HowExpert.com/books</u> – HowExpert Books
- <u>HowExpert.com/products</u> – HowExpert Products
- <u>HowExpert.com/courses</u> – HowExpert Courses
- <u>HowExpert.com/clothing</u> – HowExpert Clothing
- <u>HowExpert.com/membership</u> – Learn All Topics from A to Z by Real Experts.
- <u>HowExpert.com/affiliates</u> – HowExpert Affiliate Program
- <u>HowExpert.com/jobs</u> – HowExpert Jobs
- <u>HowExpert.com/writers</u> – Write About Your #1 Passion/Knowledge/Expertise.
- <u>YouTube.com/HowExpert</u> – Subscribe to HowExpert YouTube.
- <u>Instagram.com/HowExpert</u> – Follow HowExpert on Instagram.
- <u>Facebook.com/HowExpert</u> – Follow HowExpert on Facebook.